Magnesium

Learn About the Health Benefit of Magnesium

(Happiness & More With the Miracle Mineral Magnesium)

Rusty Adams

Published By **Phil Dawson**

Rusty Adams

*Magnesium: Learn About the Health Benefit of
Magnesium (Happiness & More With the Miracle
Mineral Magnesium)*

ISBN   978-1-77485-693-2

Legal & Disclaimer

The information contained in this ebook is not designed to replace or take the place of any form of medicine or professional medical advice. The information in this ebook has been provided for educational & entertainment purposes only.

The information contained in this book has been compiled from sources deemed reliable, and it is accurate to the best of the Author's knowledge; however, the Author cannot guarantee its accuracy and validity and cannot be held liable for any errors or omissions. Changes are periodically made to this book. You must consult your doctor or get professional medical advice before using any of the suggested remedies, techniques, or information in this book.

Upon using the information contained in this book, you agree to hold harmless the Author from and against any damages, costs, and expenses, including any legal fees potentially resulting from the application of any of the information provided by this guide. This disclaimer applies to any damages or injury caused by the use and application, whether directly or indirectly, of any advice or information presented, whether for breach of contract, tort, negligence, personal injury, criminal intent, or under any other cause of action.

You agree to accept all risks of using the information presented inside this book. You need to consult a professional medical practitioner in order to ensure you are both able and healthy enough to participate in this program.

TABLE OF CONTENTS

INTRODUCTION

How do you begin when you're trying to discuss something that has numerous advantages for your body that you can't leave bed without it? A substance that, without it the body will be on a never-ending downward trajectory, not into the earth and down beneath the earth? Something that has such huge benefits for one of the most well-known minerals that a lack of it means that other minerals are ineffective? I'm not sure what you are thinking about, but I'm talking about magnesium, the previously unnoticed star of the medical and health worlds and the mineral that can make your life hell if aren't in the right place and heaven if you possess it. Magnesium is everything and more.

Discussion and understanding of magnesium may have taken a backseat the duration that minerals, health, and medicinal concerns have been discussed however the mineral cannot be put on the backbench. Inability to recognize the good works happening doesn't mean the good works go away. It was not acknowledged however the significance of magnesium has never diminished until someplace, a person realized how vital this mineral was and began preaching the gospel.

In this book, I'll be discussing the factors that make magnesium what it is today. the miraculous mineral you ought to have abundantly in your body. The once unheard of superstar to whom all the world's focus is now to magnesium in all its glory.

CHAPTER 1: THE STORY OF MAGNESIUM

Magnesium is among the most vital minerals within the body of human beings. It is abundant throughout the body and the natural environment. It plays a vital and vital role in the minute-by- tiny functions of the body in such a way that a lack of mineral could cause an deterioration of organ systems that we recognize them. In order to ensure the efficient functioning of all organs and systems of our body, magnesium needs to be supplied with sufficient amounts daily to ensure that the body receives enough nutrients. Every day that when the body isn't supplied with sufficient magnesium could result in negative effects.

Given the significance of the mineral that we have in our bodies, it's an unfortunate fact that the majority of people are unaware of about it, or prefer not to pay attention to it. The majority of doctors do not consider the importance of magnesium and ignore it as if they don't have it. If a person is lacking in magnesium, the majority of their physicians do not do a single test. The most alarming part is that the majority of them don't even know how to determine the presence or absence, of magnesium opting to use the unreliable magnesium test, or even being aware of the issue. Doctors are aware, based on the numerous publications published that a large proportion of the world population is deficient in magnesium, but without an attempts to address the issue, we're going nowhere.

In this case that the burden falls on everyone to take care of their individual magnesium issues. You have the option of burying one's head into the sand, and avoid magnesium as some people do but you could also start the process of learning more about it and possibly to save your life or the life of somebody else. Implementation is crucial here and there's no one else that can help you gain more magnesium when your body is in need of it, other than yourself.

The mineral is plentiful in seawater and abundant in our bodies. it is the 9th highest-yielding element. It is present naturally in significant quantities for nutrition in many of the natural foods we consume. It is the most important element in human metabolism as well as an essential cofactor in more than 300 enzymatic systems which regulate our body's diverse biochemical reactions such as nerve and muscle functions blood pressure regulation glucose control, blood glycolysis control, glucose control, and the production of energy. It is responsible for sustaining the development of bones throughout existence and is essential to stabilize DNA and RNA as well as of glutathione which is an antioxidant. Since magnesium acts as a cofactor the enzymes by themselves cannot perform what they need to do with magnesium. This causes a stop to many reactions, or hinders them.

Our bodies' relationship with magnesium is a love- story of hate. Our bodies require magnesium to ensure the proper functioning of many of its organs . For it to function without problem, enough magnesium needs to be in the body. If everything is working exactly as it should be the body loses significant amounts of magnesium due to normal processes like urination and sweating. If something goes wrong and, for whatever reason, there isn't enough magnesium to allow the body to use according to its needs and health issues begin to appear.

When health issues begin to increase, the cycle is more tense than ever due to the fact that some of the medicines that you are advised to take to treat the problem could interact the magnesium levels in your body, making it disappear faster or making it useless regardless, the taking a variety of medications can cause rather than addressing the problem in hand, because the more they contribute to the destruction of the mineral the more the mineral is able to fight back, bringing on new ailments.

Magnesium is a mineral with a cellular and molecular function , which means it affects every system of our body. This is an important ion found in the body and thus utilized in chemical reactions that are fundamental within the cells of the body. It is absorbed by the body, and then circulated throughout the body using blood as the transportation channel. The blood cells utilize magnesium to carry out the routine tasks of the body and perform functions such as energy production and hormone production and maintenance of cells, as well as general movement of the body.

The effects of magnesium on the body may be as powerful as prescription medications, but the benefit of magnesium over these is that the body can recognize magnesium as its own. When it is in adequate supply it is able to be stored within bones, ready to use later on.

The numerous functions that magnesium plays in the body means that magnesium must be constantly provided in the body. It is required continuously. Inducing a relaxation in the daily magnesium supply to the body can make it difficult to remove the magnesium found in bones to the blood stream or let the body function with magnesium deficiency. There isn't a better choice between the two since the body's deficiency causes various other problems, however the loss of magnesium from bones to the blood stream implies that bones are exposed and prone to softening and weakening of bones ailments.

Therefore, it is sad that the majority of the population on earth has an insufficient amount of magnesium within their body, considering its essentiality. We eat badly, we cook food until the minerals are gone further needed, we use techniques for destroying minerals in agriculture and we take medications which are harmful to minerals such as magnesium. We damage our internal health by elevating certain minerals while ignoring others that are vital to the purpose of the increased ones. And, we consume and drink foods that cause rapid elimination of the magnesium that is present within our bodies. It's a wonder that we're still standing as a species.

The following list is the daily recommended intake of magnesium in the diet recommended by the Food and Nutrition Board of the Institute of Medicine in 1997.

Pediatric

* Infants, from birth until the age of 6 (30 mg)

* Infants, 6-months to one-year (75 mg)

* Children from 1 to 3 years old (80 mg)

* Children from 4 to 8 years old (130 mg)

* Children, ranging from 9 to 13 years old (240 mg)

* Male adolescents, aged 14-18 years (410 mg)

* Females who are adolescents, aged 14-18 years (360 mg)

Adults

* Males, ranging from 19 to 30 years old (400 mg)

* Females, between 19-30 years old (310 mg)

* Males who are 31 or over (420 mg)

* Females aged 31 and over (320 mg)

* Females who are pregnant but younger than 18 years old (400 mg)

* Females pregnant from 19-30 years old (350 mg)

* Pregnant females from 31 to 50 (360 mg)

* Females who breastfeed less than 18, (360 mg)

* Females breastfeeding between 19 and 30 years old (310 mg)

* Females breast feeding between 31 and 50 years old (320 mg)

However, you are encouraged to boost your daily intake of magnesium in times of protein synthesis that is high, like during pregnancy, during vigorous workouts, or when recovering from illness.

The only downside to the whole situation of magnesium deficiency is the difficulty in finding the levels of magnesium in the body. The test for magnesium checking blood samples for the level of magnesium present in the body is not effective since it only accounts to magnesium levels in blood at that moment and does not include magnesium in the bones or inside the cells, where the bulk of magnesium is present. This renders it ineffective and not reliable.

There is a higher chance of magnesium deficiency when:

* Experienced prolonged bouts of diarrhea or vomiting due to the fact that this causes loss of fluids from your body and consequently loss of magnesium and other minerals.

* Are suffering from digestive disorders like pancreatitis or IBS that last for prolonged periods. The condition can lead to having low levels of magnesium.

If you drink alcohol to excess, you're susceptible to magnesium deficiency due to the inadequate magnesium bioavailability. Additionally the fact that drinking too much alcohol results in frequent urination that decreases the magnesium level in your body.

If you suffer from medical conditions like diabetes, kidney disease Crohn's disease, diabetes or high thyroid levels, you're at risk of having magnesium deficiencies. The degree of deficiency will be determined by the medical situation.

* Are you prone to drinking coffee, sodas and salt to excess and this causes a decline in magnesium bioavailability within the body.

If you're taking medication such as diuretics as well as antibiotics, asthma medication estrogen pills, and some painkillers, you're at risk as these drugs result in an impairment of absorption of magnesium. In some cases these medications cause an increase in the excretion of magnesium via urine.

* Experience long and heavy period, as when you shed excessively blood from your period Certain minerals can also be lost , and magnesium may also be lost in this way.

If you are one of the people who sweat so much that you may find your clothes wet from sweat? loss of fluids in your body can result in low levels of magnesium as it's lost via sweat.

* Are you an older adult due to the fact that as an adult, you are able to have less magnesium in

your diet as compared to younger people. Furthermore that as you get older the capacity of your gut to absorb magnesium declines and the rate at which your kidneys are excreting magnesium increases and this leads to less magnesium levels in the body.

There are numerous advantages of magnesium within the body. due to this fact, there are numerous indicators that your body is able to tell that it is not getting enough of the mineral. Most organs of the body are able to are dependent on magnesium as well. There is also a great chance that whatever health issue you may be experiencing issues with, the source of your issue is due to magnesium deficiencies in your body. Watch out for signs your body might be showing. Here is an inventory of signs:

Muscle tightens and twitches

They could be the first symptoms of magnesium deficiency inside your body since the majority of magnesium is stored in tissues. Thus, these movements are the first sign that everything is not going well.

Diabetes

It could indicate the magnesium level in your body is low. Magnesium has been believed to boost the efficiency of insulin and, consequently, decreases blood sugar. However the absence of magnesium could cause insulin resistance that causes an increase in insulin. This is the source of a type of diabetes.

Insomnia

It is a neurological indication that magnesium is deficient. Magnesium reduces neuronal activity within the brain. It reduces electrical transmission between brain cells, thus making it easier to block the signals that can cause sleepiness. Sleeplessness could be the consequence of the restless leg syndrome. It is an indication that magnesium deficiencies. Magnesium deficiencies cause nerves firing at a rapid rate, which makes the brain more active to fall asleep.

Irritability

If you're feeling stressed It could be the body's way to inform you of the lack of magnesium. A sufficient amount of magnesium keeps your mind at ease because it has the ability to relax. Insufficient amounts of magnesium causes nerves to become easily stimulated.

Anxiety

This is a sign that magnesium is deficient. Magnesium can slow down the neuronal activity that occur in brain cells. It blocks the electrical transmission between brain cells, thereby making it easier to reduce the signals that trigger anxiety.

Headaches and migraines

Could be an indication the magnesium level in your body is not sufficient since when they are adequate that the magnesium present within your body is capable of stabilizing blood vessel walls and boost circulation of blood to the brain, which will protect you from migraines.

Constipation

Magnesium is a natural laxative that allows it to enhance the movement of your bowels for best and lessen constipation. It boosts the level of water in your intestinal tract, which helps to start peristalsis. Constipation can indicate that there isn't enough magnesium levels to relax the fecal matter, making an easier process for stool to move.

Sensitivity to loud sounds

Magnesium plays a crucial role in more than 300 reactions that occur in the human body. As an outcome, a deficiency in magnesium could cause various health issues such as the sensitivity to sounds. If there is a deficiency of magnesium within the body, nerves can respond too quickly to even the tiniest of triggers.

Fibromyalgia

Magnesium is known to restrain or control several nerve receptors, that have been identified as the source for a variety of forms of fibromyalgia pain. Nerves can fire excessively when there isn't enough magnesium.

Osteoporosis

Magnesium is vital for bone development and bone strength. A lack of magnesium can cause the bones becoming soft which makes them weak.

Chronic fatigue

Magnesium plays a crucial role as a co-factor in hundreds of enzyme reactions that occur within the human body. therefore the absence of magnesium could cause a variety of health issues, which include tempering with chemical reactions that affect energy production. Without this the body is unable to replenish its energy levels to help combat fatigue.

Asthma

There appears to be an association between high levels of noradrenaline as well as low magnesium levels . With asthma being linked to the high levels of noradrenaline. This may be the reason that insufficient levels of magnesium can trigger asthma. It is could also be the reason that emergency asthma attacks can be slowed by a dose magnesium.

Kidney stones

Kidney stones can be painful condition that is caused by calcium accumulation in the body. If magnesium levels are not sufficient the body's calcium may form negative alliances. in the case of kidney stones, calcium is a component of oxalate that can make hard deposits inside the kidneys. By increasing the amount of magnesium in your body, you will help treat this debilitating the condition.

Irritable bowel syndrome

Irritable bowel disease is the presence of foreign substance in your body that could be the result of toxins from the food we eat or from the surroundings. Magnesium plays a role in this since a sufficient amount of magnesium within the body is able to aid the body in detoxifying and cleanse the body of harmful poisons before they cause harm. IBS may be an indication of a deficiency in magnesium within the body.

Palpitations

It is possible that palpitations are caused by an insufficient contraction of the smooth muscle, as well as the imbalance between magnesium and calcium and more specifically a lack of magnesium, which is necessary for the preservation of healthy muscle and nerve functions.

Angina

The benefits of magnesium in the case of angina can be attributed to its capacity to enhance the production of energy within the heart and dilate coronary arteries, which results in a better oxygen supply for the heart. Angina could be a sign of low levels of magnesium within the body because of the lack of the mentioned advantages of magnesium within the body.

Reflux

The presence of sufficient magnesium in the body can be determined by the proper neutralization of stomach acid. In the absence of proper magnesium levels thus, stomach acid-related problems such as reflux and indigestion are a common occurrence.

Dysphagia

This is when you experience difficulty swallowing, and could be a sign of the deficiency in magnesium within your body. It is among the symptoms that are known to be associated with magnesium deficiency that results from the impaired the contraction of the smooth muscle which is in this instance, that is the muscles of your throat.

The amount of magnesium deficiency symptoms is a clear indication of the significance of this mineral within our bodies. It is involved in a variety of aspects and is involved in many more to perform its functions efficiently. It's beneficial to keep in mind, and be sure that you have sufficient magnesium within your body. The knowledge you gain could save your life or the life of someone else close to you.

CHAPTER 3: MAGNESIUM AS WELL AS THE HUMAN BODY

Magnesium is among the six minerals essential to comprise 99 percent of our body's mineral content. Magnesium's benefits to your body can be so vast and vast that it is hard to believe that one mineral could be able to touch all the areas of our body, however this is exactly what happens. Here is a listing of ways magnesium functions in the human body:

* It regulates the production of cholesterol.

The enzyme regulates metabolism of various nutrients such as carbohydrates, proteins as well as fats, nucleic acid and fatty acids.

* It aids in the development of teeth and fetal bones . It also aids in the growth and development of bones in infant children.

* It assists in controlling the levels of insulin in blood which reduces the risk of developing diseases such as diabetes.

* It ensures the structure of membranes of cells all over the body which allows them to function properly.

* The usage of minerals like calcium within the body are aided by the proper quantities of magnesium.

19

* It aids in the creation of energy by controlling cellular activity.

* It is a water-retention properties that facilitate stool movement, and thus treat constipation as well as other digestive tract problems.

* It helps during childbirth by decreasing the pain of labour and assists in the overall health maintenance for both mother and baby in the course of the pregnancy.

* It helps strengthen teeth and bones by aiding in maintaining mineral levels such as zinc, calcium and copper that lower the risk of weak and under-developed bones. This is which can lead to osteoporosis.

It is essential to relax muscles which is essential for the overall health of your heart. The irregularity of heartbeats can lead to tension. This is where magnesium can help to limit the heart from being exposed to different heart diseases, such as irregular heartbeats.

* Helps with DNA transcription into RNA as well as in the synthesis of proteins

Helps to relieve back pain by relaxing muscles in the back. It also helps alleviate cramps by decreasing stress in the kidney.

* Allows nerves to relay messages through the nervous system and brain to the body overall.

* Magnesium can have an euphoric effect that could be beneficial for those who suffer from anxiety or panic attacks, as well as those who have excessive stress levels.

The presence of sufficient magnesium in your body could assist in preventing bladder issues such as frequent urinary frequency.

* Magnesium is vital for adequate hydration for the body, which lets the magnesium as well as other vitamins to perform efficiently. Can help to cleanse the epidermis and cleanse skin. It also helps treat skin partsthat are prone to allergic reactions.

* Containing anti-aging properties to diminish those unwanted wrinkles and lines around your eyes.

Magnesium is a mineral that can reduce acne spots.

* It helps in healthy hair growth by forming hair follicles with strength and strong hair strands, which will stand the tests of time.

Magnesium relaxes muscle and stops the build-up of lactic acid up. This allows you to be better able and flexible.

This regulates hormone of sleep called melatonin to help you get more restful sleep.

* Magnesium deficiency causes decay of teeth and damaged teeth due to the unbalance of calcium and phosphorus within saliva.

* Plays a significant part in maintaining the strength of the immune system most notably by keeping some illnesses at the horizon.

The benefits go far beyond than this, but it provides a glimpse into the significance. It seems that there is nothing that happens in our bodies that does not tie the magnesium atom; and this is exactly what happens. Magnesium may not be the most important mineral of choice, but it is among the most vital and it is not difficult to prove that.

It's a fascinating fact that a lot of medical professionals don't consider the significance of magnesium in the plethora of health issues they encounter however, a large portion in the health emergencies they're faced with in ERs are controlled through the use of magnesium in one or another form. Here's a sample.

* Injectable as magnesium sulphate for managing seizures that are caused by toxemia during pregnancy.

* Used, as magnesium sulphate to reduce the pressure on the uterus, in order to prevent premature labour contractions in preeclampsia.

* Used to reduce the risk of convulsions during the initial treatments which lead to medical procedures.

* Magnesium intravenous has been successfully used to treat irregular heartbeats in medical procedures

Patients with constipation are treated with magnesia milk or liquid citrate to flush the bowels.

* Intravenous magnesium is utilized to treat acute asthma in patients from all ages, as it soothes the

23

airways and works as a bronchodilator. It can be lifesaving after standard treatments have been unsuccessful.

Magnesium sulphate could play significant roles for the management of acute strokes, and in reducing the chance of damage to the brain.

* It is used as a first-line medication in cases of cardiac arrest in addition to usual medical interventions.

* Magnesium Sulphate has been employed as a substitute in the event of respiratory distress.

* It reduces the tension in the smooth muscle that dilates arteries reduces blood pressure.

* May be utilized as intravenous magnesium injection to stop arrhythmias in the ventricular region that are caused by loss of electrolytes from intense training.

Additionally magnesium has also been used successfully in a variety of medical, but not in emergency room scenarios such as the ones below.

Oral magnesium can help lessen the severity and frequency of headaches, migraines, and migraines.

Vitamin B6 and magnesium can decrease the frequency from kidney stones to as high as 90 percent

* Chronic fatigue can be successfully treated with either intravenous or injection magnesium

* It could help save your life during the event of a heart attack when it is administered right after the heart attack.

* It can be used to reduce or even stop heart palpitations.

* Can be used successfully to reduce the incidence of hypersensitivity to loud sounds as well as hypersensitivity towards light.

Magnesium has proven efficient in reducing, and sometimes completely eliminating the symptoms of fibromyalgia.

* Magnesium is also successfully used to get rid of stomach acids, which can result in gastro-intestinal disorders.

* Magnesium borate, magnesium Sulphate and magnesium salicylate can be used to treat cuts and wounds.

* Research suggests that magnesium can help ease symptoms that are associated with PMS including weight gain, bloating, fatigue, and tenderness in the breasts.

* Magnesium has been utilized to prevent or reduce permanent or temporary hearing loss due to loud noises.

While some of the situations listed aren't emergency room scenarios but the importance of magnesium in those circumstances cannot be questioned. The fact that magnesium is a commonly ignored mineral that is used in such a variety of situations of life and death is almost a complete marvel. A person has described the significance for this stone as being the Holy Grail of minerals. It's apt.

The magnesium mineral has an affectionate connection with us, but this kind of relationship is an area of specialization for magnesium because it appears to be similarly with medical fields.

While magnesium is often regarded as a hero in the fight against serious medical issues There are some medications that could hinder its effectiveness or have a limited effectiveness or blocked by the use of magnesium within the body, for instance:

Antibiotics

Magnesium supplements must be taken at least an hour prior to or after taking tetracycline , macrodandin and quinolone antibiotics. The body's magnesium decreases the effectiveness of taking in these forms of medicines, including minocycline, doxycycline, ciprofloxacin moxifloxacin, tetracycline and moxifloxaci.

Calcium channel blockers

The risk and adverse side adverse effects (e.g. dizziness and fluid retention) of calcium channel blockers for pregnant women can be increased due to being in the vicinity of magnesium. Blockers of calcium channels include nifedepine felodipine, and verapamil.

Digoxin

The magnesium supplement could be needed for patients who are taking digoxin due to the negative effects of digoxin are known to cause negative effects. Insufficient levels of magnesium in blood may cause heart palpitations and nausea. However, digoxin may cause loss of magnesium via urine.

Hydration pills (Diuretics)

Certain water pills could cause a decrease in magnesium levels. As a result of this the doctors who prescribe these medicines may need to prescribe magnesium supplements to help ensure that the levels are balanced.

Penicillamine

This medication is that is used to treat Wilson's Disease and Rheumatoid Arthritis. The medication may render the magnesium's effect on the body less effective, especially when the medication is utilized for a long time. However using magnesium along with other minerals can reduce adverse effects of the drug. A doctor can tell whether magnesium supplements are the best choice for you.

Tiludronate and alendronate

They are used for the treatment or prevention of osteoporosis. Their absorption is impeded by magnesium. As a result magnesium, or antacids that contain the mineral must be consumed within an hour or two prior to the time the medication can be consumed.

Everyone needs to be aware of this information as it could help save your life or the lives of others. It is essential to be aware of when we're getting the most beneficial results from nature's bounty and also be aware of the times when everything isn't or may not be as it should be so we can be ready. It's beneficial to know the most important aspects of our lives, and magnesium is among the most vital.

It is well known that humans suffer from low levels of magnesium inside our bodies has been established. We don't recognize is the cause which cause this deplorable condition. This chapter is designed to explain the reasons for low magnesium levels and in the process, to let people know that alternative solutions are available and sacrifices can be made to ensure a steady intake of magnesium in the body in all instances.

No or low magnesium diets

Foods we consume are predominantly made from extremely processed substances that contain all the goodness, nutrients, and minerals sucked out when the process. As if that wasn't enough, an excessive intake of processed foods such as white sugar boosts the absorption of magnesium from the kidneys, which reduces the amount of magnesium that's available. Our diets are built on saturated fats that are high in saturated that reduce intake of magnesium by the digestive tract. There are foods that we consume, that contain phosphate, such as certain carbonated drinks that everyone loves however phosphates can bind magnesium, making it unusable to the human body. In addition, we aren't taking in enough magnesium the body as we could but the food we consume is trying to reduce the amount of magnesium in the body or working to decrease the amount of magnesium in the body.

Acid-forming food items

Certain foods we consume, such as white flour coffee, white sugar and sodas, as well as the alcohol we love so much are acid-forming and decrease levels of blood P.H levels. They also hinder magnesium, or other minerals to enter in the human body.

Soft water

Mineral-rich water doesn't usually have the same sweetness as water we typically would like to drink. The cows who did not drink the magnesium-rich water in Epsom did not drink it because it didn't taste good however the health benefits that came from that same water soon became apparent. However, there is no idea if the water you're drinking is high in magnesium or even contains a level of magnesium , unless you take the time to determine. Softening the water used for drinking is done to enhance the cleansing properties of water, however this procedure drastically decreases the amounts of magnesium present that are present in water. Determine whether the water you drink daily is rich in magnesium which is 10 to 30 percent in RDA for every 2 milliliters. If it isn't then you and your family need to increase your daily dosage of magnesium in order to stay as fit and healthy as you are supposed to be.

Minerals are not absorbed well by the intestine.

If your intestines are acidic it could affect your capacity to absorb minerals generally and magnesium specifically. The most common view follows that the more acidic your intestines' walls are will be, the less effective in magnesium absorption.

Calcium

This is a beneficial mineral for our body. From a very young age the children of most regions in the world learn that the lack levels of calcium within the human body contributes to weak teeth and bones. It is a fact that cannot be denied and the efforts are indeed very worthy, the one issue is that many or all of these children don't learn about magnesium for the bulk all their life. This is unfortunate as magnesium is essential to initiate Vitamin A use in the body, which aids in activating calcium usage. If you don't have enough magnesium any calcium supplements that you consume will benefit your bones. What you're actually doing is increasing the body's demand of magnesium. This is increased due to an excess of calcium. Calcium is not absorbed effectively without sufficient magnesium within the body. It is therefore important to consume these supplements in equal quantities since they function in tandem.

Medicines

The different medications we use are also battling hard to render the body's use of magnesium ineffective. Diuretics, painkillers, antibiotics, and other drugs that we use reduce the amount of magnesium in our body because they hinder the way it is absorbed or increasing the amount excreted by the kidneys.

Alcohol

Consumption of alcohol or absorption in the body could result in magnesium deficiency. Alcohol is the primary cause of liver disease which causes a decrease in quantities of magnesium. The excretion rate is multiplied by drinking or is drunk and this causes a massive removal of magnesium.

Age, stress, and illness

If you're stressed, demands for magnesium in your body are likely to rise, and cause a deficiency. Additionally, stress lowers stomach acid levels and consequently reduces the body's capacity to breakdown magnesium-rich foods and nutrients into forms the body can take in. The aging process also reduces amounts of stomach acid. The absorption rate of magnesium is contingent on the general health of the person. It's a vicious scenario in reality Low magnesium levels can result in sickness, and when you're sick, your body's inability to absorb the magnesium in the body. The main point is that magnesium is required within your body in sufficient amounts.

Salt

A majority of people in the world consume refined table salt that is devoid of nutrients. There are as many as 72 micronutrients and macronutrients which are present in sea salt. All are essential to the maintenance of health for our bodies. But, when salt is cleaned and refined most minerals are eliminated. The refined salt blocks from the absorption process of vitamins as well as vital minerals in grains and vegetables and, as a result, magnesium is also removed. However the consumption of a lot of salt can result in lower magnesium bioavailability and consequent loss or waste from the mineral.

Depleted soil

Modern farming practices have made the soils that our plants are growing mineral-free because of the frequent fertilizers that are added to the soil. Natural minerals disappear and if you do not fertilize the soil applying the same fertilizers, the food products that grow there, as fresh however they appear, are deficient of vital minerals such as magnesium and potassium.

Excessive mineral excretion

There are various processes within our bodies that cause mineral loss. Processes like sweating excessively in saunas or during sports bleeding that is triggered by menstrual issues can lead to loss of magnesium from your body. If you suffer from frequent diarrhea, magnesium may be lost in this way. When fluids are pumped out of the body in any method, magnesium and other minerals also get thrown out.

The detoxification process

The cofactors magnesium and potassium are that are required by the liver in order to rid the body of toxic substances. In a normal, healthy environment it should be simple however in the present environment of a lot of toxins in the environment as well as the food we consume the simple enzyme processes could exhaust all magnesium and potassium reserves in the body, leaving it deficient.

While the majority of methods by which magnesium is lost or is rendered useless in our bodies are beyond the control of us, there exist a few methods that, if we pay attention to and alter when it is possible to do so significant changes will be evident in our overall health. It is not possible to continue scouring as if you're in the dark after your eyes are opened. The knowledge you gain is powerful and, in this instance, it's something you should not afford to let slip by.

SUPPLEMENTS

There may be a point where you realize that the only way to absorb enough magnesium into your body is via supplements. A thing to keep in your mind is that magnesium will always be bound to other substances so you won't receive a supplement that will give the full amount of magnesium. Some supplements contain 12 40, 50, 60 or more magnesium, while those with a lower amount could offer a higher degree of absorption. The impact on magnesium is that the other ingredient might provide slightly less benefits than you would expect as well as affecting your absorption as well as its bioavailability. Here are a list of commonly used magnesium supplements that are available to you, but you'll find that some contain greater levels of magnesium, and some with very low levels.

Since magnesium is not readily absorbable by the body on itself, it needs to be bonded to a transporting chemical first and many supplement companies have consequently been chelated (ensured that the ingredient is not able to separate from digestion) magnesium into amino acids , or organic acids. The bioavailability of a product is the quantity of magnesium in the supplement. This magnesium can be absorbed , and then integrated into the digestive system , and effective in enhancing cellular function.

* Magnesium Taurate is a supplement that contains magnesium and amino acid, taurine. It has a moderate or low magnesium content, but boasts a higher degree of bioavailability. The supplement can help calm your body and mind.

* Magnesium citrate is a mixture of citric acid and magnesium. It is a laxative ingredient.

* Magnesium carbonate is a moderate proportion of magnesium at up to 45%. The supplement has anti-acid properties.

* Magnesium Glycinate is a chelated version of magnesium. It offers the most efficient absorption and bioavailability. It's the most effective for those seeking to correct the deficiency in magnesium even though it has a moderate to low magnesium levels.

* Magnesium oxide can be described as a type of magnesium that is not chelated that is bound by one of two organic acids or an fatty acid. It is awash with 60 percent magnesium, and the ability to soften stool, however it creates an acidic magnesium hydroxide inside the body that has properties that may cause burns to the walls of the intestines.

* Magnesium chloride , one the supplements that has the lowest levels of magnesium, at 12.2%, but it does have the benefit of having a greater absorption rate than other supplements.

* Magnesium Hydroxide (commonly magnesium milk) is a simple to overdose supplement that is used mostly for laxative purposes. It is crucial to adhere to the directions strictly to avoid any accidents.

Magnesium threonate is the newest child on the block of supplements. The main benefit over other supplements is its capability to penetrate the mitochondrial membrane.

* Magnesium amino acid chelate

* Liquid colloidal magnesium

Magnesium orotate is one of the most efficient magnesium supplementation forms. It is produced by using orotic acid mineral salts. Its efficacy lies due to the fact plants and animals utilize orotates for the creation of DNA and RNA.

* Magnesium lactate contains moderate magnesium levels but has the bioavailability is high in comparison to other supplements that have a higher concentrations like magnesium oxide. It is mainly utilized to treat digestive issues.

* Magnesium Sulfate is commonly called Epsom Salt. This is an organic version of magnesium that has a magnesium content of 10% but not having the greater level of bioavailability that magnesium lactate has. It is a mixture of oxygen, sulfer, and magnesium.

The non-chelated kind of magnesium that is bound to the organic acid, or fat acid. It has 60% magnesium concentration and also has properties that soften stool. The biggest drawback when it comes to competitors is that it creates caustic magnesium hydroxide inside the body, with properties that could cause damage to the walls of the intestines.

* Magnesium malate can be described as an inorganic form of magnesium that is chelated. It is believed to have one of the most efficient levels of absorption and bioavailability. It's considered to be as one of the top choices supplements for people who wish to correct a deficiency in magnesium even though it is a moderate to low levels of magnesium. It comes with a range of applications, but none are more effective than the supplements mentioned above.

* It is vital to consult with a medical professional prior to taking all of these substances. magnesium's health benefits within your body are numerous however, ensuring that your body is getting this vital mineral in a responsible manner

which includes consultations whenever they are required, like the case is for you require a doctor's guidance on the dosage of supplements.

CHAPTER 7: IT IS TIME TO HELP OUR BODIES:

MAGNESIUM-IZE

If magnesium is constantly being removed from our bodies, and is removed from our bodies and may be too little so why not take action and implement strategies to ensure you are getting magnesium into the body. It's no longer a being a case of adopting the back bencher approach and waiting to determine whether you'll experience magnesium deficiencies symptoms or not. Get active and implement the ideas that will help you get magnesium in your body either by hook or by hook or. Here are some tips to consider:

Take advantage of the treatment for magnesium deficiency.

Consuming foods that are rich in magnesium is something you should not ignore because it has positive health benefits. The milk and meat we consume contain only a tiny amount of magnesium, and the white flour, sodas, and white sugar contain nearly none. Below is a list food items that have the highest levels of magnesium.

* Chopped spinach

* Kelp

* Almonds

* Oat bran

* Brown rice

* Lima beans

* Swiss Chard

* Brazil nuts

* Molasses

* Millet

* Pecan nuts

* Cashew nuts

* Avocado

* Bananas

* Kale

Apply magnesium oil or lotions on your skin

There are many different things within your body, which are battling against taking magnesium. consequently, it is much easier to absorb magnesium through the skin than to be absorbed by the body. Therefore, it is essential for you to apply magnesium-based lotions and oils on your skin for the purpose to boost the amount that magnesium is bioavailable. The best part is that you can create the magnesium oils yourself using recipes and ingredients accessible through the Internet.

Take Epsom salt baths

Epsom salts are in fact magnesium sulfate. They earned the name Epsom because of the area in which they were first discovered. A Epsom salt bath can facilitate the absorption of magnesium through your skin, which in turn enhances the amount of magnesium within your body.

Make sure you are taking magnesium supplements that are top-quality.

Magnesium supplements contain high doses of magnesium. In the form of supplements magnesium is linked to another substance, so you cannot find a product that will give 100% magnesium. The effects on magnesium are that other substances may offer slightly different benefits than the ones expected. It could influence its absorption as well as its bioavailability. Certain supplements could provide greater amounts of magnesium, while those with lower percentages may be more absorbent. Supplements can interfere with medication or other health conditions, therefore it is essential to talk with your physician regarding the supplements you could take when you are able to use supplements.

Beware of the use of magnesium:

* Cooking can strip minerals that are found in mineral-rich food items. Consuming as many raw food as you can can help you absorb the minerals found in the food items. Consume raw vegetables along with seeds and nuts. If you must cook your vegetables, cook them at a moderate heat and don't allow them to cook for long, as this can help to reduce mineral loss.

The majority of non-organic soils for farming suffer from mineral deficiencies resulting from regular use of herbicides pesticides and fungicides that take away the soil's essential minerals.

Avoid long times of tension. Try to be a bit more stressed since stress drains the physique of magnesium.

* Reduce or eliminate alcohol as it can cause loss of magnesium due to the frequent urinary frequency.

Examine the magnesium levels in the water you consume in your community If it's lower than the level required, add a supplement.

Avoid high saturated fats as they hinder magnesium absorption in the intestines, and deplete the magnesium that is already present in your body.

* If you're on an a gluten-free diet you must take additional steps to ensure you're getting sufficient magnesium intake in your daily diet since typically gluten-free diets are known to be low in magnesium.

Take nutrients, which help magnesium

Certain nutrients assist in the process of utilizing magnesium in the body. certain nutrients also aid in its getting absorption and some aid in keeping its presence in our bodies. having these nutrients abundantly present in your body can help in keeping the proper levels of magnesium within your body. The essential nutrients are vitamins B1 (thiamine) and B6 Vitamin D3, Vitamin E, and selenium.

Take a dip in the ocean

If you live close to the ocean, or are located near an ocean, take to swim in the ocean. Sea water is so rich in amounts of magnesium., when you go swimming in the sea it gets absorbed into your your skin. This is one of the best ways to get any magnesium in your body since the rate of absorption is greater than the magnesium you take from supplements and food.

Do it organically

If it's possible you can grow your own vegetables to ensure they're produced organically. You could even raise chickens that you rear and feed so you can know what was in it. A few of the products in the supermarket advertise that they are organic, But do you actually have any method to know the quality of their organic ingredients? If you grow your own ones, you can know exactly the ingredients you are putting into the soil, so you can be 100% certain that all magnesium and other minerals are not sucked out of the soil. Of course , if you can't choose to grow your own garden or choose organic options in the supermarkets. They might not be the most efficient, but they are 50% more efficient, isn't it?

Of all the suggestions There is likely to be a few that are suitable for you. It is not necessary to take a drastic turn however, a gentle turn will get you on the right path and in no time, the ways of living that encourage high magnesium levels are element of your lifestyle; isn't this an ideal habit to establish?

CHAPTER 8: COMMON WICCAN GROUPS

Before you can become an official Wiccan You must be accepted into the coven. In the ceremony of initiation an High Priest or High Priestess isoints you to become an official member. If you don't want to join any particular coven, you may do it on your own. You can perform self-dedication ceremonies to anoint yourself.

Initiation is one of the most important aspects of Wicca. It is a symbol of the rebirth. Since the time you first accepted to the faith, you commit your life to divinities and gods. In the future, if you wish to become an High Priest or High priestess you will need to attain the Third Degree rank. You can achieve this by studying the religion.

In Wicca there are a variety of covens or groups with various practices. When you are initiated, you must select the group you would like to join. These are the most popular Wiccan groups:

* AXANDRIAN WICCA

It was created in the late 1980s by Alex along with Maxine Sanders. It puts an emphasis on the dual nature of the genders of male and female. It is associated with rites that are dedicated to the God and Goddess. The group usually meets on new and full moons. They also gather on Sabbats. If you'd like to join in this community, then you need start as a novice before moving on towards the Second Degree.

* BRITISH TRADITIONAL WICCA

They are renowned for its lineage as well as their practice and teachings and has covens throughout the globe. If you wish to be a part of this community, you must be officially initiated by an ordained linegaed member.

* Blue Star Witchcrafter

The members of the group are known as Witches instead of Wiccans. In contrast to other Wiccan groups, this one has five levels of induction. If you are interested in becoming an active member, you need to be initiated, and you must pass all levels.

* CIRCLE SANCTUARY

The Wicca Foundation is a nonprofit, religious organisation that was established around 1974, in 1974 by Selena Fox. It utilizes networking to market its own organization as well as Wicca generally. The group's members frequently hold events, like events like the Pagan Spirit Gathering.

* COVENANT OF GODESS

It was founded in the 70's and, just like British Traditional Wicca, it has several covens across various parts of the globe. The members of the coven hold annual conferences. They teach others to perform rituals, teach others about the religion, and are involved in outreach activities. They also assist people to get to know Wicca and witchcraft more thoroughly by dispelling misconceptions regarding the religion. They also offer grants and legal assistance to those who are eligible.

* Dianic WICCA

It was established in the year 2000 by Zsuzsanna Budapest and was initially able to exclusively accept women as members. In recent years, however it is beginning accepting men as members to provide the coven a polarity. Though its members are devoted to God and Goddess They are more likely to be with Goddess. They also celebrate each of the 8 Sabbats. They also permit the practice of magick that is negative including hexing cursing, and binding to anyone who harms women.

* ECLECTIC WICCA

It's a reference to NeoWiccan practices that don't belong to any particular classification. Certain covens as well as solitary Wiccans are a good example. are eclectic in their approach. Wiccans who change or adhere to diverse beliefs are known as eclectic. Furthermore those who develop their own customs are known as eclectic.

* GARDNERIAN WICCA

It was created during the 50s, in the 1950s by Gerald Gardner. The members of the coven do not seek new members. Members who wish to join the coven have to be initiated and sign an oath to not reveal to anyone outside the coven what they have experienced inside the group. If you decide to join this coven, you will only be able to read the Book of Shadows once you have completed the initative.

* SEAX WICA

It was established on the 23rd of July 1973 Raymond Buckland and was based on Saxon Paganism. It is a democratic organization that lets members choose their High Priest and High Priestess. They are also able to alter rituals and rituals that are traditional. Seax Wica does not involve any initiation rituals. Therefore, if you wish to join Seax Wica, you simply have to commit your life to the path.

The Book of Shadows

The Book of Shadows is one of the most essential tools of Wicca. It is a collection of rituals and spells that both you and the members of your group can use. The content is handwritten or computerized, however the majority of Wiccan practices recommend that it be written in hand. You can also copy from the Book of Shadows of your coven, but you could also write your own.

If you decide to create the personal Book of Shadows, make sure you have an unfilled book. If you don't have one, just bind a few blank pages together. It is possible to use any type of material to create making your Book of Shadows, but it is strongly recommended that you select materials with a sturdy construction to ensure that it doesn't get damaged easily.

In rituals using candles is an inevitable part of rituals. Therefore, it is important to be sure to protect the Book of Shadows from candle drips by covering it in an extra sheet protector. It is also recommended to include a title on the front cover. Make sure to include your name so that people are able to easily recognize the book as yours.

In terms of the content, you're free to include anything that is comfortable for you. You can also use the language that feels the most comfortable for you, for instance, the spoken word or slang. Of course, you need to add the rules that govern your group in the Book of Shadows. Each group has its own rules.

If you're a single practitioner, but your group isn't governed by established rules in writing, then you could make up your own rules. Note down what you believe is acceptable and reasonable. Make sure you establish boundaries that prevent you from going over the limit. Wiccans are expected to be accountable and disciplined.

You could also add your Wiccan Rede, your copy of the ceremony for initiation and the names of gods and goddesses that you typically use in your rituals and the reasons you have to choose these gods. Don't limit yourself to a couple of phrases or pages. You are free to write whatever you'd like inside the Book of Shadows.

Furthermore, you should note down the stones, herbs and crystals your coven makes use of. It is also important to note moon phases as well as the colors that symbolize the elements. All of this information should be placed in a table of correspondence, so it is easy to utilize them to spellcast.

Keep in mind that some spells may only be used on specific moon times. Additionally, certain spells can only be effective when the correct kind of ingredient and quantity are utilized. It is essential to ensure that you have the correct stones, crystals, or plants for your spell. To avoid confusion, make sure to see for yourself to add specific information about the elements you choose to use.

It is possible to request members of your coven to help in writing these particulars. As a novice ensure that you take note of their properties and their history. Find out if they're safe to ingest. Certain herbs should only be applied topically, and they are harmful when consumed.

It is also possible to include recipes into the Book of Shadows. These recipes can be useful on Sabbats. You can use the recipes from your coven or even find them on the Internet. You may also alter the recipes when the ingredients aren't readily available at your locale or you believe you need to alter the proportions. It is also possible to record the equipment and tools you will use in your rituals.

You can also record Sabbats in your Book of Shadows. Sabbats within the Book of Shadows so you will be informed of the dates, rituals, and many other aspects. This Wheel of the Year consists of eight major Sabbats. They are Samhain, Imbolc, Yule, Litha, Ostara, Beltane, Lughnasadh, and Mabon. Certain traditions don't celebrate the eight Sabbats.

If your coven is one that celebrates an evening of full moons, it is possible to add Esbat as a ritual in the Book of Shadows. It's up to you whether you would like to use the same ritual for each ritual, or choose a new one for each. Include details about the casting of a circle, Drawing down the Moon or other rituals to heal or protection and wealth. It is possible to include Astrology, Tarot and scrying.

Maintain the Book of Shadows as detailed and filled with information as you can. Note down the steps you completed and the results you've gotten. Don't forget to note down ancient prayers, sacred text and chants. You can translate prayers into English or write them down in the original languages.

Ideally, you'll need separate books for your spells as they may be quite a bit to include into your Book of Shadows. The use of a separate book to store your spells makes them more organized and easy to locate. If you don't utilize many spells or want to keep the spells in your Book of Shadows, you might want to do that too.

When casting spells, make sure to record the particulars. You may note down the results you obtained. This will allow you to determine which spells work to your advantage and which don't. You can stop using spells that don't work and use the ones that work.

Remember this: you are using the Book of Shadows is a sacred instrument. You must take great attention to it. You should not ignore it. It is also essential to keep it updated with the contents as often as you need to. If you do not wish to be able to do it with difficulty updating it, tie the pages with rings bounders. This will allow you to easily add additional pages whenever you need to.

Dividers can also be used to help make your pages more organized. Also, ensure that you have an Table of Contents that you regularly update when you add more information to the Book of Shadows. A Table of Contents will allow you to discover the spells or the information you need faster and easily.

It is the Phases of the Moon

The moon's cycles are essential for the practice of magick. Wiccans are of the belief that the moon is magical in its properties, and its different phases may result in different results. Therefore, it is crucial that you plan your activities in accordance with the moon's phases.

THE WAXING MOON

The phase changes from dark to full , and generally takes 14 days to complete the cycle. In several Wiccan practices positive magick is performed during the time when it is the time of waxing moon. They seek to attract positive energy and make themselves better. In this period you may do rituals to improve your love, money, career and objects.

Waxing Crescent Moon Crescent Moon

It is often referred to by the name of Moon of Regeneration, and is anywhere from 45 to 90@ ahead of sun. In this period, you are able to plan your future and gather information, establish an outline, or start to change your life. Also, you can prepare for your life's goals. The crescent moon or the waxing crescent moon is the ideal time to reenergize. In this period, strengthening your body and strengthening it are the most effective since you are able to absorb both the positive and negative energies more efficiently.

1st Quarter or Waxing Moon

It is also called it is also called the Moon of Caution, and ranges from 90 to 135@ before the Sun. It lasts between 7 and 10 1/2 days following it is the full moon. In this period it is it is the Time of Warrior Maiden is observed. The theme is represented through Artemis, Minerva, Athena, Diana, and Bridget. It is the ideal time to be able to feel intuition, intuition and energy. Also, it is the best time to do renewal and rejuvenation.

Waxing Gibbous Moon

It is often referred to by the name of Moon of Endings, and is 135 or 180@ more than the Sun. At this time the greater part of the moon's light is provided by the sun. This is the best moment to tie up loose ends and get ready for the energy that will come from the full moon.

THE FULL MOON

It is often referred to by the name of Moon of Celebration and is between 180 and 255 miles over the Sun. At this moment, the entire face that the moon faces is clearly visible. Wiccans are known to perform spells at times when the moon's at its full since they believe it is the time when it is most effective. They typically do their rituals for three days, which includes the day prior and the day following. Some groups have their members be able to base their rituals on different phases of the moon.

Full moons are the appropriate opportunity to make spells to help with spiritual and personal development. It's also the perfect time to be carrying out any significant work. It is possible to cast healing spells and spells to increasing your magical abilities and psychic awareness. Additionally, you can use spells to bring you feel closer to gods. Additionally, you can do the Esbat ritual.

THE NEW MOON

It is often referred to by the name of Dark Moon as well as the Moon of Rest and Beginnings. In this period it's right within the solar system and earth, which is the reason it's not visible. This is the only period that solar eclipses is visible. The moon is the range of 0 to 45 degrees over the sun.

In the period of the new moon, you are able to make spells to bring new beginnings and ventures. It's the best moment to relax, find new affection, develop in gratitude, and re-energize. It's also the ideal time to let go of negative habits. Furthermore, it's the ideal time to begin new initiatives.

The time of the new moon is the time when you see the fruits of your efforts. It can also be somewhat difficult to carry out work during this time since the moon is not visible. A lot of Wiccans believe that the new moon as a time of fallow, during which they relax and refuel before performing more intensive activities. Some Wiccans are, however, inclined to view the new moon to be an opportunity to do magick associated with granting wishes.

THE MOON WANING

It changes from full to dark and remains that for about two weeks. At this time it is a symbol of goddesses as Crone and is thus the most suitable for deep insight and divination. Wiccans typically perform a shamanistic ritual during the time of waning moon. They seek to get rid of the evil, demolish, and take away everything they don't need anymore.

The last night of the moon is the ideal moment to cast spells to getting rid of bad behavior or relationships or getting rid of an employment position, or for reducing the burden of debt and other negative aspects. It's also the ideal moment to let go and safeguard yourself from people and influencers who are negative to you.

Waning Gibbous or disseminating Moon

It is often referred to by the name of Moon of Retribution or the Moon of the Earth Mothers which is located approximately 225 to 270° in front of the sun. At this time it is the best time to look over actions, rectify mistakes, resolve disputes and amend any mistakes. Wiccans connect the moon's waxing to everyday issues. They also believe it is a catalyst for growth in the human spirit.

The Last Quarter, or the Waning Moon Moon

It is sometimes referred to also as the Moon of Harvest, and ranges from 270@ to 315@ in front of the sun. It is ideal for getting rid of negative energy and ending certain patterns and relationships. At this point you should eliminate everything that creates obstruction. This is the ideal opportunity to take a break, relax to recuperate, prepare to release the energy released through the full moon.

Magnesium is fourth in the list of the fourth most abundant mineral in the human body. About 99% of the Magnesium found in the body is intracellular and only 1% found in the extracellular area. The distribution of the body Magnesium is as following: 60% of Magnesium is located inside bones. The remaining 20% is found in the heart's cells and muscles , and 19% can be found in the soft tissues and the liver.

It would be easier for the body to have the capability to create Magnesium on its own , but this isn't the case. The mineral is available to the body through the oral ingestion (food as well as supplements) and parenteral methods (intramuscular intravenous, intravenous, or intravenous infusion) or through transdermal or topical administration.

Foods rich in Magnesium

The positive side is that there is a wide variety of cheap, tasty, and easily accessible food items that are high in Magnesium. They include:

* Deep, green leafy vegetables. Examples include kale, infant spinach, collard greens , and Swiss Chard.

61

* Fruits like avocados, bananas , and dried Apricots.

* Fish. This includes tuna, halibut wild salmon, mackerel and wild salmon.

* Nuts such as cashews Pecans Brazil nutsand pine almonds and nuts.

* Seeds. Examples include flaxseeds, pumpkin seeds and sunflower seeds.

* Beans and peas like chickpeas, lentils, black-eyed peas kidney beans, white and black beans.

* Soy-based products like tofu and tofu.

* Whole grains, such as brown rice and millet.

* Plain yogurt that is non-fat

* Dark chocolate

How is it that deficiency can still occur even though oral intake of Magnesium rich foods is sufficient? The problem is that Magnesium in these foods can be diminished through processing and poor cooking. Additionally that, the body can only absorb about 20-50 percent of Magnesium due to problems with digestion and renal excretion. Therefore, more sources are required.

Magnesium supplements

It's not uncommon that numerous primary health professionals recommend Magnesium supplements to increase the levels of this mineral within the body. But there are many differences in the supplements available. Magnesium supplements are the same. So, you must be cautious in your selection of supplements. Take into consideration the following aspects:

1. The absorption capacity and solubility that the ingredients have.

2. What food should you include with the supplements in order to maximize bioavailability (the percentage of the supplement that gets into the bloodstream to create the desired effects).

3. It is the compatibility between selected supplement to one's digestive system.

While the recommended dose in the recommended dosage of Magnesium in adults lies 300-400 mg per day many nutritionists and doctors suggest at least 500 mg or higher doses to people who suffer from diabetes, alcoholism depressed, or on an pharmacological treatment for diuretics or anti-cancer medications in particular Cisplatin. But, patients suffering from kidney disease cannot use Magnesium supplementation (even the minimal dose) without consultation and guidance from their physician.

The presence of diarrhea can serve as indication that they are taking too much Magnesium. If this is the case one simply has to reduce the dosage that the mineral is taking until it ceases in its tracks. For people who suffer from constipation but, Magnesium is the answer to their issue.

Magnesium for Parenteral Use

Magnesium Sulfate injections can be used to control and treat immediate signs of life-threatening diseases like severe toxemias and acute Nephritis (among children) as well as hypomagnesemia that is accompanied by symptoms of tetany, as well as those who are receiving parenteral nutrition.

Be extremely cautious prior to the administration of parenteral Magnesium Sulfate. Follow these steps to ensure the security for the person receiving it.

1. First, check your blood pressure. Do not test if blood pressure is extremely low.

2. Test for knee-jerk reflexes. Do not test if they are not present.

3. Create a dose IV Calcium Gluconate to counteract.

4. Examine the pulse and respiratory rate. Do not administer if the respiration rate is 12-breaths-per-minute or lower, and the pulse is less than 60 beats per minute.

5. Check if patient can void.

Topical Magnesium Topical

Magnesium can be absorbed transdermally (thru to the surface). There are creams, lotions, and sprays available in pharmacies. It is also possible to get this amazing mineral while bathing or into Magnesium salts.

The benefits of transdermal or topical Magnesium as compared to supplementation or eating Magnesium-rich food items are as follows:

• They're more affordable, convenient and efficient. They are also safer.

* They have less negative side effects.

Results are instantaneous because diffusion of ions occurs more rapid via the skin then the digestive tract. It takes around 20 minutes.

* There is no risk of overdosing with the topical Magnesium since the skin absorbs only the necessary amount.

* It's safe for pet and children. Mix it with water in baths.

Magnesium oil has also become more and more popular in recent times. It's not really oil in itself, however it appears and feels similar to oil. There are complaints of rashes and discomfort in the initial few days of use, however this is simply a sign that the person is lacking in Magnesium. The best method is dilute the oil with water from a spring or purified water source and then apply small amounts on the legs and arms. After a few days, you can apply the oil over the entire body.

To increase the absorption of Magnesium through the skin, the following activities are possible to implement:

1. Expand the area of application. It's been discovered that the armpits and scalp are more absorbent in comparison to other body parts.

2. Increase the time that the topical treatment is applied to the skin.

3. Increase the number of times of applications.

4. Increase the temperature of the area of application , as research has shown that the more warm the application area, the more absorbable it will be.

5. Hydrate your skin since there is a faster absorption when skin is properly hydrated.

A lack of magnesium can cause an illness known as hypomagnesemia, which is a condition that causes a lack of magnesium within the body. In the next section discover the symptoms and signs, the tests and treatments for hypomagnesemia.

Hypomagnesemia: Signs and the Symptoms, Tests and Treatment

Hypomagnesemia occurs when the blood concentration of Magnesium is lower than 1.5-2.5 mEq/L. There are instances of a higher blood concentration of Magnesium (hypermagnesemia) but these are uncommon and likely to be caused by overdoses of supplements or the administration of parenteral medication. Hypomagnesemia is quite widespread and it is estimated that 70 percent of the population are suffering from it.

The causes of hypomagnesemia

Apart from insufficient intake and inadequate absorption of Magnesium Deficiency can be caused due to:

1. Stress

2. Alcoholism

3. Chronic diarrhea

4. Malnutrition

5. Malabsorption disorders, such as intestinal inflammation

6. Certain medicines. Examples include aminoglycoside antibiotics proton pump inhibitors, anticancer and diuretics medications.

7. EXCESSIVE URINATION

8. Other MEDICAL disorders, such as HYPERCALCEMIA and HYPERALDOSTERONISM

9. Profound sweating

10. 2nd and 3rd degree burns

Affects and Signs of Hypomagnesemia

The severity that you have Magnesium deficiency, patients suffering from hypomagnesemia might be afflicted with the following symptoms.

Mild deficiency Magnesium

• Loss of appetite, also known as anorexia

* Weakness or fatigue

* Apathy

* Confused

* Trouble sleeping

* Irritability

* A reduced ability to learn

* Poor memory

* Lethargy

Moderate deficiency in Magnesium

* Rapid heartbeat

* Changes in the cardiovascular system

*Tetany (positive positive for Chvostek and Trousseau sign hyperreflexia, carpopedal spontaneous spasm)

Severe deficiency in Magnesium

* Delirium

* Tingling sensation

* Hallucinations

* Number

* Continued muscle contraction

* Convulsions

Hypomagnesemia-related complications

* Respiratory arrest

* Cardiac arrest

* Death

The symptoms are treatable through treatment. In addition the prognosis of hypomagnesemia is usually excellent, particularly when it is treated and diagnosed promptly.

Conditions that are a result of a deficiency of Magnesium

There are many diseases which could be caused directly or indirectly by an imbalance in the Magnesium blood levels. Here are a few:

1. Allergies

2. Alzheimer's Disease

3. Arthritis

4. Asthma

5. Back back pain

6. Hypertension

7. DIABETES

8. CANCER

9. Cerebral palsy

10. Kidney stones

11. Liver Cirrhosis

12. Pancreatitis

13. Parkinson's disease

14. Tetanus

15. Stroke

16. Varicose veins

17. Disorders of the mood (bipolar, depression and anxiety)

18. OSTEOPOROSIS

19. Poor memory

20. Capacity to learn is reduced.

Tests to determine if you have hypomagnesemia

The doctor can request the following lab tests and diagnostic tests to check for hypomagnesemia

1. Blood test for Magnesium

2. Blood test for calcium

3. Potassium level

4. Comprehensive metabolic panel

5. Urine magnesium test

6. Electrocardiogram

Treatment for Hypomagnesemia

Based on the severity of the deficiencies, patients could be treated with Magnesium via parenteral, oral or transdermal ways. Doctors can additionally prescribe calcium and Potassium supplements since hypermagnesemia may result in low levels of potassium and calcium.

The most important thing is the bottom line

There is no way to survive without Magnesium. The advantages of having a sufficient levels of Magnesium within the body are too numerous to take for as a given. But there are risks that deficiencies can be deadly. The proper Magnesium level is essential.

THE CARDIOVASCULAR BENEFITS OF MAGNESIUM

One of the main advantages of Magnesium is the health of your heart. Around 20% of the body Magnesium is located in the heart's cells and muscles. Insufficient levels can cause atherosclerosis as well as congestive heart failure. chest pain, hypertension cardiomyopathy, cardiac arrhythmias (heart muscular disease) heart attack, and, eventually, death. What causes this?

The role that Magnesium throughout the cardiac system

1. Regulates potassium-sodium exchange pump. In the past, the significance of Magnesium in the control of electrolytes has been highlighted. With

regard to heart health, it's well-known that potassium is essential to the heart's functions. A deficiency in this electrolyte could lead to heart arrhythmias. Magnesium plays a role in maintaining the balance between exchange of sodium and potassium. If there is a deficiency in Magnesium the cells are unable of cells to store potassium, resulting in the depletion of potassium in the intracellular space. This could lead to abrupt cardiac deaths. Only after correction of the Magnesium deficit will potassium deficiency be corrected as well.

2. Influences blood circulation. Circulation is severely affected when there is hypomagnesemia. In addition to the endocrine tissues that have vasodilation the rest suffer from vasoconstriction resulting from calcium entry into cells and prostaglandin synthesizing. It is due to a lack of Magnesium which is the key ingredient in control of Calcium. Insufficient circulation to the heart could result in ischemia that may lead to myocardial infarction , and ultimately to cardiac arrest.

3. This prevents the development of atheroma. Studies have revealed that a lack in Magnesium is associated with the malfunction of the endothelium in the arteries, hypercoagulation of blood, and a higher the concentration of lipids. The three causes are all contributing to the

progression of atherosclerosis. In addition that hypomagnesemia can lead to vasoconstriction, which can further aggravate the condition. If the deficiencies are not rectified, it could be fatal for the person affected.

4. Inhibits the coagulation factor. Magnesium is also involved in increasing the prothrombin time (how long blood clots last). Furthermore, the formation of platelets is also slowed through Magnesium. In addition, the formation of thrombuses is reduced or prevented too. This decreases the possibility of blockages forming along blood vessels' walls.

5. Relaxes muscles. The tight and tight muscles cause a decrease in circulation, which increases the blood flow pressure across the walls of arterial. Without Magnesium muscle cells would remain contracted. The muscles are relaxed and there is no cramps happen in the presence of a sufficient quantity of Magnesium. Furthermore, pain in the muscles would be reduced as well since with the presence of this miraculous mineral, the build-up of lactic acid up will not occur.

Food to think about

Because of these roles in the heart it is easy to see the importance Magnesium is for the heart. The majority of the time it is taken for granted.

It is false to believe that taking Magnesium is the sole key to an ideal heart. There isn't a shortcut to this. A healthy lifestyle is vital. If one looks at the issue more closely it is possible to see the connection between Magnesium and an active lifestyle with a heart that is healthy.

Magnesium and lifestyle modification equal healthy heart

Alcohol consumption, for instance, can cause the depletion of Magnesium. This is why it is important to stay clear of drinking alcohol. It will not just protect the liver, but also the GI tract and the other vital organs, but also the heart as well.

Another change in lifestyle that is necessary is to stop smoking. Smoking is a bad habit that makes you an ideal potential candidate to be a victim of Magnesium deficiency. How? Smoking causes blood cholesterol levels to increase and the Magnesium level drops. Both can result in heart problems.

Living a lifestyle that is sedentary does not seem to be linked to Magnesium deficiency , but there is no. As mentioned earlier, Magnesium promotes conversion of glucose into energy units. Inactivity could cause sugar to accumulate instead of used. The glucose stored would turn into the fats that are accumulating within the body in the future. It's been proven that being overweight or obese can result in a myriad of heart diseases. It is therefore more beneficial to put the energy you have in productive activities like exercise and strength training.

Sleep deprivation has many drawbacks. The connection between insomnia and a low Magnesium level has been confirmed through various research studies. Thus, an adequate consumption of Magnesium will eliminate this harmful habit and , at while, help improve the health of your heart.

Stress is a factor in almost all heart-related diseases. Many people are unaware that stress can result in Magnesium depletion. Therefore, it is important to be able to manage stress in a way that you can avoid heart disease and Magnesium deficiencies (which can cause heart disease also) and thus ensures the health of your heart.

Magnesium's benefits to the heart

The heart is among the most vital organs of the human body. A healthy heart can lead on the following

* Longer life

* More energy

* Lower risk of developing numerous medical ailments

* A boost in mood

* A stronger respiratory system

* Lessening the risk of cancer

* Improved neurological functions

To summarize the point is that there is a greater quality of life offered to people with healthy hearts. So it is essential. It is possible to achieve this by making sure that is getting enough Magnesium. To improve the health of your heart, a change in lifestyle is essential, too.

The Relationship between Magnesium and Happiness

A lot of people are unable to recognize the connection with Magnesium and their personal happiness. It's true that there are many elements which contribute to a feeling of happiness. However, if you eliminate Magnesium from the equation, and depression, as well as other mood disorders will develop. It's an established fact. Happiness is contingent on Magnesium as well.

What are the causes of happiness?

Happiness is a matter of personal preference. What may be happiness for one person may not be a happy experience for someone else. Studying happiness shows the various reasons why that people feel happy and happy. These are the reasons why Magnesium is a major factor. Here are a few of them:

1. Neurochemicals. The body produces a variety of neurochemicals. Magnesium enhances its production of neurochemicals. Thus magnesium, neurochemicals, and happiness can be a pair. The neurochemicals that are linked to happiness include:

It is a. Dopamine, also known as the reward chemical. When a person succeeds in achieving an objective it is a feeling of satisfaction. This is due to an increase in dopamine levels within the brain. Thus, occasions of triumph or success provide a feeling of joy.

B. OXYTOCIN or the BONDING MOLECULE. This is the NEUROCHEMICAL RESPONSIBLE for HUMAN BONDING. When there is an attachment whether it is a man-made or not in NATURE, THE PERCENTAGE OF OXYTOCIN released is increased. In turn, there is an increased level of JOY and satisfaction that is felt. Studies also revealed that human touch, intimacy, lovemaking and AFFECTATION CAN INCREASE levels of OXYTOCIN. Pet owners can also experience a higher level of OXYTOCIN, if they bond with the animals.

C. Endorphins, also known as the pain-killing molecules. The body craves pleasures , not suffering. There is a profound feeling of joy when you are free of discomfort. Endorphins are released when a person is engaged in physically demanding activities such as strength training or sexual interactions.

D. Serotonin or the confidence molecule. If you have an appropriate amount of self-esteem, self-worth and self-confidence, happiness also exists.

E. GABA or the anti-anxiety chemical. GABA provides the sensation of calm and peace. The absence of tension and anxiety is a sign of happiness for some people.

F. Adrenaline is the energy molecules. Adrenaline is a chemical that makes you feel alert energetic, excited and alive. It provides the energy needed to complete numerous things.

2. Hormones. Certain hormones may cause people to feel happy or bad. For instance when one is stressed the stress hormone cortisol releases. Research suggests that the lower levels of cortisol can bring a sense of happiness to people. Magnesium plays an important function in the control and regulation of different hormones.

3. Physical health. As we mentioned previously, Magnesium contribute a lot to the overall health of the heart as well as other organs that are vital to our health. If one is physically healthy and

happy, they have a higher sense of well-being and also happiness.

4. Health and emotional wellbeing. It is all about the emotions. Sadness and happiness are both manifestations of emotion. Through the use of Magnesium people are able to tend to be content. The effects of sedation from Magnesium help to calm and manage emotional outbursts , while the excitation effects can make people positive and enthusiastic. Both can lead to happiness.

5. Health and social. Happiness is in part with how you interact to others, too. In addition to regulating hormones and stimulating neurochemicals creation, Magnesium provides increased energy levels. These factors can lead people to be more physically active and more social. The prevention of anxiety, depression suicidal tendencies, depression and various mood problems has been linked to the proper amount of Magnesium within the body too.

6. Mental health. Magnesium also improves brain functions. There are numerous pleasures from having a higher mental health. Happiness can also be achieved when an individual is comfortable with his mental well-being.

Miracle Remedies Using Magnesium

Magnesium isn't only enough to be called the "Miracle Mineral" but also of a variety of adjectives like incredible, amazing, phenomenal, and magnificent. It is worthy of being recognized and acknowledged. Its positive effects on one's heart well-being, happiness and overall wellbeing are incredibly beneficial. But, there's more!

Many are unaware that Magnesium may also be the solution to these aforementioned problems.

1. Age-related effects. Magnesium's properties make it possible to combat the effects of ageing including weakened immune system and increased risk of chronic illnesses, and a decrease of energy. It is possible to age gracefully and still live a full life. Magnesium has the ability to prevent the any occurrence of age-related ailments. These diseases have been found to decrease physical activity and affect mood. They also alter brain function and decrease the length of life. Research has shown that Magnesium can slow down the process of aging. How? The rapid aging process has been linked with a disproportionate shortening of Telomeres. They are the tips that protect of the chromosomes. Afficient Magnesium levels can stop the telomeres from shortening.

2. Obesity and overweight. Man has been fighting this problem since the beginning of time.

Magnesium is a powerful antioxidant that fights weight gain by three methods:

a. It assists the body in its ability to absorb, digest and use the fats ingested as well as carbohydrates, proteins and. It's a well-known fact that improper use of these substances may cause the body to store glucose and fats that encourage the growth of abdominal fats and various regions of the body.

b. It plays a significant ROLE in the CHEMICAL REACTION between GLUCOSE AND INSULIN. When a PERSON is consuming FOOD it is when the BODY converts it to the GLUCOSE. To allow GLUCOSE to be utilized it has to enter the cells. But, like a key to a door INSULIN is needed for the GLUCOSE to get into the cells. Without INSULIN, GLUCOSE WILL REMAIN OUTSIDE and that's where the blood GLUCOSE LEVEL is lowered. The BODY is still hungry, even the fact that GLUCOSE is available. MAGNESIUM STOPS THIS FROM HAPPENING AS IT PROMOTES INSULIN SENSITIVITY. This stops the elimination of both INSULIN and GLUCOSE levels. Thus, the unnecessary cravings for CARBOHYDRATES and the need to consume food are reduced. This is how DIABETES is also promoted.

C. It reduces the negative effect of stress. Stress and obesity are linked for a long time and for a variety of reasons. When you are stressed the hormone cortisol gets released. The increase in cortisol levels puts the body on alert, and appetite is diminished as the body's means to "conserving" the food intake and food items in the event of an need for emergency. So, the sugars and fats aren't used up. This is only the beginning. Once when the "danger" is thought to be gone, the body will attempt to restore normalcy through increasing appetite. This causes the person to consume food even though there is no requirement to, as the calories weren't burned off in the first place. This process is repeated, which results in the weight increase. Magnesium is believed to be the primary mineral to deal with stress. It increases the neurochemicals that fight stress and boost positive mood and happiness.

3. Infertility and other issues with gynecology. Not many people know that Magnesium is a preventative for Premenstrual Syndrome, dysmenorrhea, premature contraction (among pregnant women) Preeclampsia, eclampsia, and pree. Additionally it has been proven to solve problems with infertility among females. How? Magnesium is a key component in the creation of progesterone, also referred to as "hormone that causes pregnancy". In addition, as we already mentioned, Magnesium allows delivery of nutrients and oxygen to different organs of vital importance such as the uterus, due to its effects on circulation. Be aware that Magnesium creates

vasodilation, which allows sufficient tissue perfusion.

4. Colorectal Cancer. This kind of cancer is the second most common cause of death for cancer patients, both females and males. In addition it is also the third most frequent cancer for both genders. Magnesium could be thought of as an effective strategy to prevent cancer since it lowers the chance of developing tumors in the rectal and colon regions. Research has shown up to 13% reduction in the likelihood of developing cancer of the colorectal can be achieved when there is enough Magnesium within the body. Apart from that, almost all Magnesium rich foods are high in fiber, and happen to be the diet recommended to avoid colorectal cancer.

5. Beauty. Magnesium can also be an effective natural enhancer of beauty. By utilizing Calcium as well as other mineral, Magnesium improves the health of hair and makes skin more youthful.

The final words about Magnesium

These are just a few of the amazing remedies Magnesium can offer. Magnesium is easily accessible inexpensive, safe and effective. It is truly a marvel in every sense. There is much to gain by ensuring that you have a sufficient Magnesium levels in the body. There is much at stake when someone suffers from Magnesium deficiency.

You don't have the ability of a genius realize how crucial Magnesium is for health. Make sure you are prepared to reap the numerous benefits associated from the usage of Magnesium. Make the decision now to live an enjoyable, healthier and longer life simply by taking Magnesium.

CHAPTER 10: MANGNESIUM (MG12) OVERVIEW

Magnesium is a glistening gray chemical element, and is the 8th most abundant element found on earth. Magnesium accounts for about thirteen percent of earth's total mass and an important portion of the mantle. Magnesium is created in massive older stars when three nuclei of Helium are added to carbon nuclei. When a particular star explodes, producing the phenomenon known as a supernova, the majority of magnesium is released into the interstellar space to be reused into different star systems developing. This results in magnesium being the 9th most prevalent substance in our universe. Also, magnesium is the third most abundant element found in seawater.

While magnesium is an element of the periodic table is able to be formed naturally only when it is combined with other elements. At this moment it will always be in an oxidation state of +2. While most commonly made in nature, magnesium can be manufactured. If it is made by humans magnesium is made, it is highly reactive which is why it is covered with an extremely thin coating oxide.

Magnesium is essential to the functions that the body performs since it's the 11th most abundant element in our body. The ions of the element are crucial for the proper functioning of all cells and are in contact with polyphosphate molecules like your DNA. While magnesium is an essential component to the body's functioning and structure, a lot of individuals are known to be deficient in magnesium. Magnesium's natural properties are numerous which we'll discuss in the future. However, some of the most commonly used uses for magnesium include anti-causes, as a laxative, and also to ease the symptoms of eclampsia. However, it's not the most delicious element in the world, since the ions are unpleasant to the taste. But, it is usually used in smaller amounts to give natural tartness in mineral springs.

The term "magnesium" is derived in the Greek word "magnesia," which is an area in Thessaly. The usage of magnesium is long but the most important discoveries in magnesium started in the early 1600s. A farmer from Epsom, England had tried every trick he could think of to have his cows drink water from a well, but the water tasted too bitter to cattle to drink. Through his efforts the farmer discovered that the water soothed and healed small scratches. This led to the first time that we learned about Epsom salts. This substance later identified as magnesium sulfate hydrated.

About two hundred years after, in 1808 Sir Humphry Davy first produced the in fact, magnesium-based metal. Utilizing electrolysis to create a combination of mercuric oxide and magnesia the scientist was able to make magnesium in his laboratory. The year was 1831. Antoine Bussy prepared the mineral in a stable and acceptable form.

Without magnesium our bodies would not be capable of producing energy, and muscles will remain in an inactive state. Magnesium ions play a crucial part of the creation and utilization of ATP which is the primary source of energy that is found in the cells of your body. Also, we would not be able to adjust our body's levels of cholesterol produced and released into the bloodstream. The magnesium ions participate in a myriad of biochemical reactions within the body due to their function as co-factors of enzymes. Magnesium is also essential for the balance of your mineral levels and in your body's internal processes for making proteins as well as the creation of new cells within your DNA and DNA and.

Magnesium comes in many forms Magnesium chloride can be naturally found in seawater. Magnesite is a rock that is referred to as magnesium carbonate. it is present in chlorophyll, the primary element found in the plant material.

Magnesium chloride can be the most easily absorbed and readily available type of magnesium.

The living world is comprised out of hydrogen, oxygen carbon, nitrogen and oxygen. These tiny elements are utilized to form tissues and body fluids for animals and humans. In addition to these four essential elements all the rest of your body's composition is comprised of minerals. Magnesium is macro-minerals, meaning that your body requires huge quantities of it in order to function effectively. Some of the more well-known macrominerals are potassium, sodium and calcium. All of these are included as a regular element of a balanced diet. In the average, the human body contains around twenty-five grams of magnesium. This is required to replenish every day. When you consume magnesium, it's broken down, and released to produce separate magnesium ions. In its pure form the magnesium ions are positive charge.

Magnesium and Your Health

As you've seen earlier in this chapter the magnesium mineral is an essential element that is present in the body. The mineral is responsible for and aids in a variety of crucial actions, reactions, and systems. The average adult has twenty-two and twenty-five grams of magnesium in their bodies. Sixty percent is located in the skeleton. Thirty-nine percent are found in muscle skeletal and the remaining part is extracellular. The usual levels of magnesium serum in the human body is between 0.8-1.0 mg/L. Even when levels of magnesium in the body are quite low, levels of magnesium in the serum are normal. The significance of keeping an average or higher amount of magnesium in serum is related to its role in absorption of gastrointestinal contents and the function of the kidneys.

The proper levels of magnesium can to treat and prevent many conditions and diseases, beginning with cardiovascular disease and high blood pressure. Blood pressure levels are the most significant risk factor for heart disease and stroke. Numerous studies have been conducted which have proven that when people with a high risk of stroke or heart disease, add more magnesium to their diets, it decreases the chance of suffering from heart disease or stroke.

Magnesium is among the most essential nutrients for supporting the heart and assisting it function more effectively. It also helps guard blood vessels, which is the heart disease occurs. Another method that magnesium assists in helping to prevent heart diseases is through functioning as a blood thinner similar to the actions of aspirin.

Magnesium supplements are also believed to reduce the chance to develop Type 2 Diabetes. Magnesium assists your body in breaking down sugars, thereby reducing the chance of developing insulin resistance. Insulin resistance can be a problem that contributes to the development of Type 2 Diabetes. However, there are ongoing studies underway to determine if the high amount of magnesium are effective in treating the condition. Researchers have discovered that people who suffer from diabetes have lower levels of magnesium that those who do not suffer from diabetes.

The component most often associated with healthy bones and joints is calcium. But magnesium is essential for bone health as it helps treat and stop osteoporosis. Many people choose to supplement their diet with calcium in order to build their bones. However, the problem of weak bones results from a lack of magnesium. People who consume higher amounts of magnesium are more likely to have a higher bone density. When bone density is greater, it decreases the chance of osteoporosis and fractures. It has been proven that women begin losing more bone mass than men around thirty years of age. Magnesium supplements can help to reduce and stop bone loss.

It is vital to be aware that when the magnesium levels in your body rise and the calcium levels in your body decrease, thereby preventing hypocalcemia from occurring or causing hypercalcemia. Also eating a lot of protein could hinder the absorption of magnesium. Therefore, it is essential to ensure that you're not deficient and eating sufficient foods that have large levels of magnesium. If your body is consuming excessive magnesium, it depletes the mineral through urine, feces and sweat.

More than 12 per cent of United States population suffers from migraines. Similar to bones, women are more likely to suffer from migraines than males. Numerous studies have indicated that people suffering from migraine headaches are suffering from low concentrations of magnesium present in their bloodstream and tissues. In the majority of cases that were studied the researchers discovered that magnesium supplements could help reduce the frequency of migraines. However, prior to attempting to treat migraines using magnesium supplements, you should consult with your physician to determine the root source of your headache.

Magnesium is regarded as the most effective antidote to tension and stress. It's possibly the most potent relax mineral that can aid in improving your sleep. Actually magnesium plays a crucial element in a great night's rest. Studies suggest that even a tiny lack of magnesium stops the brain from resting in the night. Magnesium helps to calm your nervous system and increases your quality of sleep.

Dymenorrhea is more often referred to as menstrual cramps, is typically caused by fluctuations in or low levels of magnesium. Menstrual pain is triggered because your body's pain receptors are stimulated by increased prostaglandin levels. Prostaglandins, or chemicals, are present found in the uterus which can cause the uterus to expand. Therefore, magnesium plays a significant role in the health of women's reproductive system. Higher doses of magnesium are able to alleviate a variety of severe and painful symptoms commonly associated with menstrual health. These include hunger, weight control infertility, cramps, and cravings. Women's magnesium levels fluctuate during the menstrual cycle due to estrogen levels are higher. the more estrogen you have and more magnesium levels are.

Magnesium is also an essential element in good digestion. The body utilizes magnesium to aid in the digestion process by controlling the levels of copper, potassium, calcium and vitamin D. Magnesium activates enzymes within the body that aid in the absorption and utilize protein, fats as well as carbohydrates. Through activating these enzymes, your body will be able to process food and break it down into energy-producing particles. The factors mentioned above are what make magnesium an essential solution for relieving constipation.

Magnesium is utilized to make neurotransmitters that aid in improving concentration and attention. It can also have a relaxing effect on the brain as well as the nervous system. This makes magnesium an ideal natural remedy to manage ADHD symptoms. In many cases, deficiency in magnesium can result in decreased concentration, a lack of concentration, and even confusion. In the event that you are or your kid is diagnosed with ADHD seek out an expert in medical care in order to establish if magnesium might be an appropriate treatment.

Magnesium is a great supplement for those struggling with obesity, similar to the way it aids patients suffering from diabetes. Even though overweight people consume large quantities of foods, they are more likely to be severely malnourished. This is due to the poor nutrition in their meals as well as in the vast array of foods that are available to us. Leptin plays a significant role in the development of obesity, however magnesium is a seldom discussed mineral that is a key factor. Research has shown the fact that when you produce significant amounts of leptin you will notice an upsurge in the amount of magnesium content in the urine of your. Type 1 diabetics suffer the most from loss of magnesium due to excessive urine. Leptin levels that are high with low levels of magnesium cause inflammation, which results in the weight gain and heart disease as well as diabetes.

To build muscle, those who train regularly are inclined to consume large quantities of protein. While protein can certainly aid in building muscle however magnesium is also essential to build strength. As you've read magnesium is the principal ingredient that aids in muscles to contract. If you don't have enough magnesium, it is impossible to develop muscles. Magnesium also plays a role in protein synthesis within the body, which helps to rebuild tissues and decreases inflammation. Insufficient magnesium levels mean that you are in a position to perform at the highest level and gain the strength you need.

MAGNESIUM DEFICIENCY

Research has shown that more than 60 percent of Americans suffer from magnesium deficiency. Magnesium plays a crucial role in the body's functioning and without it, the body's system are likely to experience extreme reactions. Even though the majority of the population is lacking in magnesium the condition is referred to as a silent epidemic. Most people do not recognize the issue and consequently is often left untreated. The diagnosis of magnesium deficiency can be very difficult. Blood tests are the most common method of assessing the level of nutrients in your body. however, only 1% of magnesium that is present that is in your body gets released into your bloodstream. This is why it's essential to recognize the signs that indicate low levels of magnesium.

Aspects Side effects of Magnesium Deficiency

* Nausea

* Vomiting

• Loss of appetite

* Weakness

* Fatigue

* Seizures

* Tingling

* Muscle Cramps

* Number

* Dysrhythmia (Irregular Heart Rate)

The diet of the majority members of people in the United States population provides less than half the recommended magnesium intake. This is a common deficiency in males older than 70 years old age, and teenagers. If a diet high in magnesium is paired with supplements to the diet the total consumption of magnesium is likely to be higher than the recommended amount.

MAGNESIUM OVERDOSE

According to the old saying "everything should be taken in moderation." It doesn't matter if it's watermelon or vitamins, eating too much of a single item can be harmful for your health. While the majority of people is lacking in magnesium, taking in too excessive amounts can result in serious harm too. If you are taking magnesium supplements and suffer from any of the signs immediately take medical advice such as swelling of the tongue, face as well as the throat and lips. Be aware of these signs:

The Side Effects

* Nausea

* Vomiting

* Flickering

* Light-headedness

* Stomach Upset

* Change in heart rate

* Tingling

* Redness under the skin

* Bloating

* Gas

* Diarrhea

Since more than 50 percent of the population are lacking in magnesium and it could be difficult to get a dose too high with the mineral. As you've read there are evidently many advantages and negatives of supplementing with magnesium. This is only the beginning of amazing things magnesium can do to improve your life. Keep reading to discover how magnesium benefits your garden and home!

Magnesium Benefits for Your Home and Garden

Magnesium isn't just beneficial for your health internally and appearance, but also your physical appearance, your home, and your garden too. It is in the form of magnesium sulfate, more popularly referred to as Epsom salts The benefits that this mineral can provide are infinite and can be utilized throughout your daily life. In this section, you'll be taught every method you can incorporate Epsom salts into your daily beauty regimen, your flower beds and even your bathroom!

HOME REMEDIES and PERSONAL Salt EPSOM USE

Removal of splinters: If have ever been the victim of an splinter, you're aware of the pain they can be. They are entangled in your skin and require cautious tweezing in order to get them out. Utilizing the simple remedy of soaking your affected area with the concentrated Epsom salt water will help pull the splinter away naturally, without any further discomfort.

Sunburn Relief: Sunburn is one of the most unwelcome moments of summer and when you are on vacation. Simple things like washing and dressing can result in intense discomfort. Aloe Vera gel is the most commonly used remedy for quick sunburn relief. However, magnesium sulfate can work just as effectively to treat minor sunburn. Use a spoonful of Epsom salt, combine it in half of a cup water. Then, refrigerate. Spray bottle to cover the burned areas to ease pain. This mixture will treat itchy bug bites as well as minor burns.

Help with Sprains and Bruising: Epsom salts are a natural and safe treatment to ease sore sprains and bruises. Magnesium Sulfate contains anti-inflammatory properties that help ease soreness.

Add two cups Epsom salts in warm bath water , and then massage your body to ease the pain.

Foot Soak The most popular ways to use Epsom salts is to add the salts to a foot bath in the water and then soak your feet. While the Epsom salt and warm water solution can aid in relieving pain and aches but it can also help combat athlete's foot as well as other fungal diseases. Simply add half 1 cup Epsom salts to the warm water in a tub and let your feet soak for however long you'd like.

The Face Scrub: Magnesium Sulfate is an excellent exfoliant for your skin and face. Exfoliating is essential to maintain your skin health since it gently cleanses away dirt and grime inside your pores to prevent your skin free of acne. All you have to add is a teaspoon of Epsom salt to cleanse your face and gently massage it onto your face in small circular movements. Rinse, and then enjoy the extra smoothness on your face.

Extra Volume in Hair: There is no need to invest a huge amount of money on costly mousse or other hair products! You can achieve all the needed volume for your hair by creating a hair mask made of Epsom salts. Mix equal amounts of Epsom salts and conditioner. Then apply the mixture to hair. Allow the solution to set in your hair for 20 minutes before washing. Allow your hair to dry naturally for long and silky locks.

SALTS FROM EPSOM INSIDE THE HOME

Cleaning Tile and Grout Epsom salts paired with dish soap create a rough solution that can scrub off even the most thick layer of dirt from the kitchen or bathroom tiles. Get rid of elbow grease and go for mixing equal amounts of Epsom salts along with dish soap liquid to make an easy-to-cleaner that will clean your property. Make sure you rinse the surfaces thoroughly by with a gentle scrub.

Washing Pans and Pots Magnesium sulfate can work just well with your dishes as it does on grime and tiles! Food residue can get accumulated and can be difficult to remove when it is ignited into metal. Instead of straining your arms muscles while scrubbing off dirty pans and pots and pans, add a few drops of Epsom salts into your dishes and aid in cleaning food particles that have accumulated. The rough structure of salts can effortlessly remove dirt without causing damage to the cookware.

Cleaning Detergent Residues: Over some time, the detergent for washing and softener residue will begin to accumulate in your dryer and washer. It is possible to use Epsom salts to remove the detergent residue and make your washing machine run more effectively. Just let the washing machine be filled with warm water. Then, add one quarter cup of white vinegar as well as one cup Epsom salts. Let the machine shake the mix for a few minutes. After that, stop the process and let the mix sit for at least an hour.

Charge your car battery It is possible to give a little more life to the battery in your car by applying a small amount of Epsom salt to its battery cells. All you have to do is add one 1 ounce of Epsom salt in the water in a cup until it completely dissolves. Add the paste to each cell of your battery and your battery will last longer. more life.

Christmas Decorations: You can make your windows appear of frosty and festive without spending a lot of money on expensive window decorations. Mix 1 and 1/2 cup of water that is boiling and 1 cup Epsom salt. After that, you can add three tablespoons of dish soap in liquid form. Utilize a sponge to add the solution onto your windows to give them a frosty appearance!

EPSOM SALT Solutions for your GARDEN

More nutritious and larger vegetables: Epsom salts work as an natural fertilizer and soil to help feed your plants. For better tasting and healthier vegetables in your backyard, simply add a teaspoon of Epsom salt in the soil under the plant to encourage growth.

House Plants House plants are difficult to manage properly. They require sun, foodand an accurate consumption of water to survive. Finding a balance between all these elements could make it difficult to decorate your home with colorful plants. If you do include a few tablespoons Epsom salt in a pot of water before you water your plants, they will flourish and bloom.

Eliminating Garden Invaders If you're not a huge bug fan Slugs are unpleasant to behold. They're slimy and gnaw at your plants, damaging your crops and flowers. Sprinkle Epsom salt on your soil will deter the weeds from taking over your flower gardens.

Take a sniff of the roses The smell of roses is like the beauty of roses that are blooming in the spring! To aid in the growth of your roses and blossom more beautifully you can add one tablespoon each week into the soil around your rose bushes before watering them to ensure an increase in growth.

The Soil Enhancement Method: Magnesium sulfurate can be used as a soil preparation for the planting of stunning flowers and veggies. Before you begin planting the garden, add two or three bags Epsom salt into the already prepared soil in your garden. Water it to increase the magnesium level of soil.

Grow greener grass: The majority times your soil will require an additional boost of iron and magnesium to keep plants healthy. For your grass to be more vibrant and greener you should add 2 tablespoons of the mixture for each gallon of water you use and spread the mix on your lawn.

Raccoon Repellent Raccoons can cause havoc to the garbage cans in your home and spill the leftover meatloaf from last week across the ground. If you've got furry visitors lurking around the house late in the evening all you have to do is sprinkle a couple of teaspoons of Epsom salt over your containers to rid them completely! Raccoons do not like the smell of salts and will be able to stay away so long as you ensure that you apply an additional layer when it rains.

Magnesium and food

You can fix your the deficiencies in magnesium by adding magnesium-rich foods into your diet. Magnesium can be found naturally in many different foodsthat can be beneficial for weight loss and establishing the ideal way of life. This is a complete list of the various foods that you can incorporate into your meals or as snacks to get more magnesium!

Food Serving Size (mg)

Almonds 14 Cup 61.64

Asparagus 1. Cup 25.20

Barley .33 Cup 81.57

Basil 1 Cup 13.57

Beets Cup 39.10 Cup 39.10

Beet Greens 1 Cup 97.92

Bell Peppers 1 Cup 11.04

Black Beans 1 Cup 120.40

Bock Choy 1 Cup 18.70

Broccoli 1 Cup 32.76

Brown Rice 1 Cup 83.85

Brussels Sprouts 1 Cup 31.20

Buckwheat 1. Cup 85.68

Cabbage 1 Cup 25.50

Cantaloupe Cup 19.20 Cup 19.20

The Cashews 1 1/4 Cup 116.80

Cauliflower 1 Cup 11.16

Celery Cup 1 Cup 11.11

Cloves 2 teaspoon. 10.88

Collard Greens 1 Cup 39.90

Cucumber Cup 1 Cup 13.52

Cumin 2 TSP. 15.37

Flaxseeds 2 tablespoons. 57.96

Green Beans 1 Cup 22.50

Green Peas 1 Cup 53.72

Kale 1 Cup 23.40

Kidney Beans 1 Cup 74.34

Lima Beans 1 Cup 80.84

Millet 1 Cup 76.56

Mustard Greens 1 Cup 18.20

Navy Beans 1 Cup 96.46

Oats 1/4 Cup 69.03

Papaya 1 Medium 57.96

Parsley Half Cup 15.20

Pinto Beans 1-cup 85.50 Cup 85.50

Pumpkin Seeds 1/4 Cup 190.92

Quinoa 3/4 Cup 118.40

Raspberries Cup 1 Cup 27.06

Romaine Lettuce 2 Cups 13.16

Scallops 4 oz. 41.96

Sesame Seeds .25 Cup 126.36

Soy Beans 1 Cup 147.92

Spinach 1 Cup 156.60

Strawberries 1 Cup 18.72

Summer Squash Cup 1 Cup 43.20

Sunflower Seeds 1/4 Cup 113.75

Tomatoes 1 Cup 19.80

Tofu 4 oz. 65.77

Tuna 4 oz. 47.63

Turnip Greens 1 Cup 31.68

Watermelon 1 Cup 15.20

1 Cup 58.24

Magnesium supplements and measuring Your Consumption

After you've read about the various food items that supply you with sufficient magnesium to meet the daily recommended dose (RDA) You may be wondering what milligrams of magnesium are you consuming each day. Fortunately, it's easy to locate charts and guidelines online that offer thorough explanations of the proper amount to meet your sexual and age. Below are straightforward, easy-to-follow instructions to make it easier for you.

Children

Children aged 1to 3 years must be taking in at least 80mg daily.

Children between 4-8 years old should consume 130 mg of vitamin C every day.

Children between 9-13 years old should consume 240 mg of a daily dose.

Females

Women aged 14-18 years old should consume 360mg of a day.

Women who are between 19-30 years old should consume 310 mg of a daily dose.

Women aged 31 or older should consume daily 320mg.

Pregnant Women

Women pregnant who are younger than 19 are advised to take 400mg of adrenergic agonists daily.

Women expecting a baby between 19-30 years receive 350mg per day.

Pregnant women who have over the age of 31 must consume 360mg of folic acid daily.

Breastfeeding Women

Women who breastfeed and are less than 19 years old should consume 360 mg of a day.

Women who breastfeed between the ages of 19 and 30 should be taking daily 310 mg.

Women who breastfeed who are aged 31 and older must take 32omg daily.

Males

Men between the age of 14-18 years must take 410 mg daily.

Men between the age of 19-30 years should consume 400 mg of the drug every day.

Aged men of 31 old or older must consume 420 mg every day.

Different Magnesium Supplements and Magnesium Types

Try to meet your daily magnesium target through food is the most secure option instead of taking supplements. The reason is that the use of supplements in excess could result in a magnesium overdose, which can be hazardous and can be fatal. But, there are many safe options of supplements that are suggested by medical professionals across the nation. Magnesium supplements are available in multivitamin-mineral pills as well as other supplements to your diet. The various kinds of supplements that provide magnesium in safe amounts include aspirate, magnesium lactate magnesium chloride as well as magnesium citrate. Magnesium can also be found in various laxatives as well as products to treat indigestion and heartburn.

If you decide to try magnesium supplements It is essential to understand all the varieties available in the market. Be aware that magnesium is only discovered in conjunction with other substances, which means there isn't a product or pill that is completely comprised of magnesium. This is to ensure that your body is able to take in the minerals and utilize it efficiently.

1. Magnesium Glycinate: This type of magnesium has the most bioavailability as well as absorption. It is believed to be the ideal supplement for people trying to get rid of the deficiency of magnesium.

2. Magnesium Oxide: The type of magnesium has a binding to fat acid. It has sixty percent magnesium, and has the ability to help the

digestive system to create a stool that is soft and more comfortable to go through.

3. Magnesium Chloride as well as Magnesium Lactate The form of the mineral is 12 percent magnesium. It is however, more readily absorbed in comparison to the other magnesium supplements such as magnesium oxide.

4. Magnesium Sulfate as well as Magnesium Hydroxide Magnesium Sulfate and Magnesium Hydroxide: These two supplements are referred to as magnesia's milk. They are typically employed as laxatives, so be aware of this before you attempt to take supplements. Be aware that these magnesium forms can be abused therefore, only take them according to the instructions of your physician.

5. Magnesium Carbonate : This form of magnesium is a antacid with properties. It also consists of 45 percent magnesium.

6. Magnesium taurate type of supplement of magnesium contains a blend of taurine and magnesium it is an amino acids. When combined with supplements, they typically have a relaxing effect on the nervous system, which can help to relax your body and mind. This makes magnesium taurate a perfect all-natural sleep supplement.

7. Magnesium Citrate: The form of magnesium also contains citric acid. Citric acid helps with the properties of laxatives.

8. Magnesium Threonate is the most advanced version of magnesium supplements. As of now, studies have revealed promising benefits. This type of magnesium is able to penetrate mitochondrial membranes to produce stronger effects. Magnesium threonate is believed to be the top mineral supplement in the market.

Caution

To ensure your wellbeing, it needs to be reiterated how harmful the consequences of an overdose on magnesium could be. Like any other supplement, drug, or vitamin, consuming excessive amounts of one substance could result in serious harm. It is essential to be cautious when trying new ingredients in your food. If you decide to go an approach of using supplements with magnesium it is more difficult to overdose, which can result in numerous uncomfortable symptoms and negative results. Get immediate help from a physician in the event that your tongue, face the lips, or throat start to become swollen.

Other side effects that are common to magnesium overdose can include and aren't limited to nausea, vomiting, fainting, lightheadedness, stomach upset and a rapid or slow heart rate, redness or tingling on your face, constipation gas and diarrhea.

Magnesium is regarded as the mineral missing from the majority of people's lives. Nearly half of people are in need of magnesium, however this does not mean you're not. Before you start taking magnesium supplements or increase your intake of magnesium-rich foods discuss with your physician to determine if it's essential to boost the amount of magnesium you have. People who are also suffering with heart or kidney disease should supplement with magnesium under medical supervision. If you're experiencing any of the signs or side effects and symptoms, you must seek advice from your doctor promptly to determine the cause.

There are many reasons that may be causing your body to be rid of excessive magnesium. Drinking excessive quantities of soda, coffee or alcohol may trigger this impact. Additionally, consuming large amounts of sugar and sodium could cause magnesium deficiency. There are a variety of prescription and medication options that can cause loss of magnesium; consequently, you should talk to your doctor if you believe this could be the reason of the magnesium deficiency. Certain of these medications could include blood pressure medications and diuretics. A rise in magnesium levels could trigger modifications in prescription drugs. It is a possible interaction with blood pressure medications and antibiotics mediation, therefore speaking to your physician is essential prior to attempt to diagnose yourself.

CHAPTER 11: IMPORTANCE OF MAGNESIUM TO WOMEN'S

HEALTH

Everyone requires magnesium for different functions in the body, such as strengthening bones, improving your mood, tackling depression, and treating respiratory issues and digestive issues. But, among both genders, women require magnesium in greater quantities than men, particularly for aiding in pregnancy, managing anxiety, headaches and PMS as well as other issues that are common among women. Let's look at why magnesium can benefit women:

Magnesium Supplements for the duration of pregnancy.

While pregnant, you require adequate magnesium levels to guard against a variety of issues like preterm birth and preeclampsia. Preeclampsia is a complication of pregnancy which affects approximately five percent of females. It is defined by hypertension. Another aspect of this condition is the damage of blood vessels in lung, kidneys the brain or liver. It could lead to multiple organ failure that is followed by convulsions and coma. death. The condition can only be cured by the birth of the infant.

Other complications associated with pregnancy that magnesium may help in preventing is poor fetal growth and infant death. It is recommended for women expecting a baby aged 19-30 years old to consume about 350 grams magnesium each daily.

Magnesium for PMS

Magnesium is utilized in many enzyme reactions that regulate functions of our brain. It can also aid in the treatment of disorders like bipolar as well as PMS. Magnesium also aids to ease muscle spasms and spasms, as well as in the production of energy , and in improving the functioning that of your heart. It is recommended to boost your magnesium intake prior to the beginning of menstrual flow to manage severe mood swings.

Lowers the Risk of Diabetes

The results of scientific research have shown that women who are overweight and taking just a tiny amount of magnesium were more vulnerable to the effects of the type II form of diabetes. The study that involved around 40000 women suggested that women need to consume more magnesium through eating foods such as fresh vegetables and almonds and supplementation.

Lowers Blood Pressure

Medical experts suggest a balanced intake of magnesium in order to lower blood pressure. Based on numerous research studies that recommend women consume a large amount of magnesium to reduce the risk of hypertension particularly during pregnancy. Why is this you might ask? Magnesium is a key component in expanding blood vessels, which reduces blood pressure to alleviate problems like preeclampsia and eclampsia. Both of these issues result in an increase in blood pressure, especially during the final trimester.

Magnesium is also proven to be effective in preventing other issues like seizures. If you're a woman with a age of 31 and over, you ought to consume 320 mg of magnesium.

Reduces leg cramps

A lot of pregnant women suffer from painful leg cramps. The problem can be avoided by a three-week intake supplementation with magnesium.

Prevents Osteoporosis

Bone health is generally improved by the consumption in Vitamin D, calcium and magnesium. Women attain their highest bone mass at the age of 18-30 years old, and after that it is a gradual decline in bone density. Menopausal women are an increase in the rate of loss of bone. Insufficient magnesium levels have been been proven to cause postmenopausal osteoporosis. This is a condition that typically occurs during the menopausal age and is marked by very porous bones that could easily break. This is caused due to the fact that a deficiency of magnesium could affect the calcium metabolism as well as the hormones that regulate calcium.

Reduces stress and prevents attacks

Have you realized that adequate magnesium can help you fight anxiety attacks and strengthen the nervous system? Alongside managing depression and insomnia magnesium can also ease other serious mental disorders, including excessive anxiety or panic attack.

Reduces the risk of Cardiovascular Diseases and Diabetes

It is advised females to consume magnesium-rich food items and supplements to reduce the risk of developing coronary heart diseases. Numerous studies on diet have found that taking adequate quantities of magnesium could reduce chances of having a stroke. However the low level of magnesium increases chances of suffering from heart attacks. So, make sure you get sufficient magnesium levels to improve your heart health.

Alongside the deficiencies of magnesium, which causes cardiovascular diseases In addition, magnesium deficiency can result in type II diabetes with severe diabetic retinal disease. This is due to the fact that magnesium an essential component of the carbohydrate metabolism, and can influence the production and functioning of insulin. Consuming around 100mg of magnesium could reduce the risk of developing diabetes by 15 percent.

I'm sure that you're aware the importance particularly for women to consume magnesium. What would happen in the event that you do not take sufficient quantities of magnesium and suffer from magnesium deficiencies?

Conditions that are Related to Magnesium Deficiency

There isn't any lab test that will establish the exact amount of magnesium within the body's tissues. This is because just 1 percent of the mineral is found in blood serum, which makes it difficult to complete the process of testing. Doctors frequently test urine tests to determine magnesium levels, however these tests show only estimates.

Typically, the amount magnesium within your body is typically measured in relation to the symptoms you are experiencing. The absence of magnesium does not cause specific symptoms, however the full-blown deficiency in magnesium may cause you to feel tired, weak and nauseous. Deficiency that is severe can lead to severe problems, including irregular heart rhythm seizures, muscle contractions, seizures as well as numbness, tingling and tingling and uncontrollable eye movements.

It is also possible to experience persistent symptoms, such as heart spasms, a condition that is characterized by a blockage of blood flow in the arteries that blood flows into the coronary. A higher magnesium deficiency can result in hypocalcemia, or low calcium, and also hypokalemia or low potassium which can be fatal. Extremely low levels of magnesium within the body could cause cardiac arrest, respiratory arrest and even the death.

These are the conditions that are caused by magnesium deficiency.

Atherosclerosis

This type of cardiovascular disease is characterised by the hardening and clogging of the arteries and blood vessels. The cause is primarily by the build-up of fatty acid deposits, or cholesterol. Insufficient amounts of magnesium could cause more harm since it can affect blood pressure, metabolism, and platelet formation. Typically, a deficiency of magnesium can result in higher levels of bad cholesterol, lower quantities of HDL or good cholesterol and higher levels of triglycerides. Magnesium consumption can reduce bad LDL cholesterol, while increasing the amount of good HDL fats.

Osteoporosis

Studies have shown that the rise in magnesium intake can improve the bone density by up to 80 percent. If you're a female suffering from postmenopausal issues you must consume at least 1000 mg of calcium per day to increase your calcium to magnesium ratio. The ideal ratio for calcium and magnesium is 1:1 however women need to consume more calcium in order to make the ratio 1:4.

Asthma

Numerous studies have shown that when you suffer from asthma the magnesium content of your body is generally low. Boosting the amount magnesium levels can ease asthma symptoms. The supplementation of magnesium has demonstrated an increase in lung activity and the capacity to circulate air into and out of lung. However low levels of magnesium can cause a worsening of asthmatic conditions and wheezing.

Most multivitamins are not formulated with magnesium because the mineral is extremely bulky and may create a tablet that is quite big. Other multivitamins contain magnesium antagonists, which assist in reducing the amount of magnesium within the body. This is the reason why continual use of multivitamins can lead to the formation of allergies and asthma.

Calcification

The condition is described as a change to the form of calcareous or stony substance due to the accumulation of calcium salt or lime. The condition can be seen within the kidney as and in heart valves. Renal calculi are defined by the influx of calcium phosphate phosphate salts within the kidney, which is an organ that filters blood and generates urine. The intake of magnesium through the mouth has proven to decrease stone formation and the urine saturation ratio. However magnesium deficiency may cause the calcification of the valves in our hearts. Consumption of magnesium via oral treatment has also been proven to lessen the effects of the disease.

Attention Deficit Disorder

Did you realize that one of the most important cause in Attention Deficit Hyperactivity Disorder (ADHD) and Attention Deficit Disorder (ADD) is magnesium deficiency? Research has proven that lack of magnesium in sufficient amounts is among the major causes of these conditions. The majority of children suffering from the two types of disorders suffer from magnesium deficiencies.

Diabetes

Magnesium deficiencies are believed to be responsible for increasing the risk of developing diabetes which is the seventh leading cause of death in Americans. The majority of people don't take in the proper amounts of magnesium and therefore are susceptible to developing the type II form of diabetes. The most effective sources of magnesium are the magnesium-rich foods since supplements and multivitamins aren't as effective for treating diabetes.

Depression and anxiety

The research shows a clear correlation between magnesium consumption as well as depression. A deficiency of this mineral is often the cause of an rise in anxiety and depression for the majority of people. Insufficient magnesium levels in the blood serum can result in increased anxiousness and increased. It is vital to understand that your body needs magnesium to carry adrenaline throughout the body for controlling hypertension and relax muscles that are contracted. Deficiency in magnesium consequently, causes tense muscles, hypertension and excessive levels of adrenaline, which contribute to hyperactivity.

Allergies

Magnesium deficiency has been linked to negative allergic reactions as well as chemical sensitivities. The condition is marked by increased scratching and redness of the skin. In the case of allergic reactions, levels of histamine as well as white blood cells are also elevated. If you suffer from chronic illnesses there is a tendency to suffer from skin allergies, an increase in white blood cell levels as well as other different types of allergies.

Based on the data gathered regarding the conditions you could be suffering from due to magnesium deficiency, it is crucial to combat magnesium deficiency. Let's see what we can do with diet to attain this.

Using Diet To Fight Magnesium Deficiency

When you recognize that you have a magnesium deficiencies, you must to take in the mineral through the whole food items that contain the mineral in its organic form. The plants contain the green-colored substance known as chlorophyll that is helpful in converting sunlight energy into energy that can be utilized for metabolic purposes. Chlorophyll is comprised of magnesium, which is an element that allows plants to absorb sunlight's energy. Green vegetables, for instance. Swiss and spinach are rich in magnesium, along with avocados and beans. Other sources include seeds and nuts, such as sunflower seeds, sesame seeds, pumpkin seeds and almonds.

While you should consume food items that are rich in magnesium you might also wish to know that certain circumstances or conditions can impact how magnesium is absorbed, and consequently, make you insufficient even after taking the food. To be sure that you're getting enough amounts, you must ensure that the following issues aren't affecting magnesium absorption and utilization. These comprise:

1. A weakened digestive system may hinder your body's capacity to absorb magnesium due to issues such as Crohn's disease, leaky gut, or Crohn's.

2. Kidneys infected by infection can cause excessive loss of magnesium via urination.

3. The condition is more severe when it is not managed, results in a loss of magnesium via urination

4. Different medications, such as diuretics, antibiotics, and diuretics are among the drugs used to treat cancer. These ailments can lead to a magnesium deficiency.

5. Alcoholism is a condition in which over 60 percent of those who drink have extremely minimal levels of magnesium

6. As we age, people are more likely to becoming magnesium deficient since the rate of absorption decreases as we the advancing years. Also, women who are older are likely to be taking more prescription medicationsthat can affect taking magnesium.

7. Candida can block your body from absorbing magnesium because higher levels of Candida in your body dissolve the Candida metabolites and turn in an insufficiency

8. An everyday drinker of caffeinated beverages, including tea, soda and coffee, because the kidneys are responsible for monitoring magnesium levels, and caffeine triggers kidneys to release magnesium regardless of health condition.

Foods with high Magnesium levels

It is recommended to manage magnesium levels via food rather than using supplements. One of the most effective methods is to eat diverse meals that include numerous dark-green leafy vegetables which are organically grown. These plants, which are fertilized, typically contain high levels of potassium, phosphorus , and nitrogen, in contrast to magnesium. This list lists the most magnesium-rich foods in relation to the magnesium content in 100 grams:

Seaweed dried that has 770 mg magnesium

Dried coriander leaf, 694 mg

Dried pumpkin seeds, which contain 535 mg

Unsweetened dry powder Cocoa of 499mg

Dried Basil with 422 mg

Ground Flaxseed, 392 mg

Almond butter, approximately 300 mg

Sweet and dried Whey with 176 mg

Below are a few foods you can pick to boost your magnesium content.

Dark Leafy Greens

They are extremely essential superfoods that provide a variety of vital minerals and vitamins, in addition to additional health advantages. Dark leafy greens are the best choices for magnesium sources because they are low in calories. The most nutritious greens to opt for are Swiss Chard, Kale, raw collared and baby spinach.

Nuts and seeds

Did you know that just half 1 cup of seeds from pumpkin provides your daily magnesium nutrition requirement? Other nuts rich in magnesium include pecans flaxseeds, pine nuts cashews Brazil nuts as well as sunflower seeds and almonds.

Fish

In addition to the abundant levels of vitamin D and omega-3 fatty acids it is recommended to include additional fish to your diet to gain magnesium. Fish such as tuna wild salmon, halibut and mackerel are rich in amounts of the mineral. Make sure you eat fish for dinner or lunch each week. Or you can try making the salmon salad.

Soybeans

It is a great source of nutrients like amino acids and vitamins as well as minerals, and also has large quantities of fiber. Soybeans provide about half of the magnesium you require daily. You should aim for a 1/2 cup serving of soybeans that have been roasted and dried as a snack, so that you can get the most benefit from these minerals. Other legumes contain high quantities of magnesium. These include chickpeas and black-eyed beans, kidney beans, white beans and black beans.

Avocado

The fruit is rich in heart-healthy nutrients as well with a variety of multivitamins. It is in fact one of the most nutritious and adaptable foods that you can eat. Add a slice of avocado to your lunchbox or transform it salad to gain 15 percent of your daily quantity of magnesium.

Bananas

Bananas are renowned for their abundance of potassium, which help build your bones stronger and improve heart health. In addition, a medium-sized banana will provide you with approximately 32 milligrams of magnesium, along with Vitamin C, as well as other fiber. This makes a banana an ideal choice for those who are trying to lose weight because it's only 100 calories and should be part of snacks or breakfast. Other fruits with significant amounts of magnesium are grapefruit, figs, strawberries, and blackberries.

Dark Chocolate

Along with its sweet flavor Dark chocolate is also an ideal choice for regular snack or dessert because it's rich in magnesium. Dark chocolate provides approximately 24 percent of the daily recommended magnesium intake and is not a high calorie food since it is only 140 calories. The dark chocolate you consume is high in antioxidants which help to ease hypertension, improve the heart's health, and increase blood circulation. You can pair dark chocolate fresh fruit for a dessert that is sweet and delicious for after-dinner.

Low-Fat Yogurt

For your body to absorb magnesium, you also need to factor in calcium as part of the nutritional content. Dairy products among them yogurt are a great source of magnesium too. A container of low or no-fat yogurt contains around 19 milligrams of magnesium. Try incorporating a fiber-rich fruit with low-fat yogurt for your breakfast.

Dietary Tips To Increase Magnesium Intake

1. Aim for more magnesium-rich meals among them veggies, nuts, and beans. Veggies are very suitable for dieters aiming to burn fat or lose weight as they contain fewer calories. Try making a soup from veggies, meat, and beans, simmer it overnight in your Crockpot and consume the following morning for breakfast.

2. Try eating healthy fats along with your diet in order to boost the absorption of nutrients.

Scientific research has proven that magnesium is easily absorbed with consumption of salad containing fat.

3. While you need to take in adequate amounts of calcium to ensure adequate absorption of magnesium, too much calcium is not good. Therefore, avoid eating too much calcium rich foods or drinking excess milk as this might lower magnesium level in the body. In addition, taking calcium in large amounts interferes with proper functioning of your heart which magnesium tries to enhance.

4. Try obtaining magnesium from dietary sources as opposed to supplements, as magnesium is an alkaline mineral. Supplementing with magnesium lowers your stomach's acidity and thus hinders nutrient absorption. You also need other minerals for proper assimilation as opposed to supplements that offer only magnesium.

5. Do not consume soy products in excess as they raise estrogen levels and thus hinder absorption and utilization of magnesium in your body. Soy foods can also result to thyroid problems and thus should be consumed in moderation.

Using Supplements To Fight Deficiency

Magnesium deficiency problems that supplements are designed to address include migraine headaches, kidney stones and hearing loss. Magnesium supplements are also believed to cure insomnia, restless leg syndrome and enhance athletic performance.

Medical experts in most circumstances may recommend you to use supplements to treat problems such as premenstrual syndrome (PMS), eclampsia, preeclampsia, hypertension or a very high level of high-density lipoprotein or bad cholesterol. You can also be required to buy magnesium supplements to address chronic conditions such as chronic fatigue syndrome, fibromyalgia, multiple sclerosis, and diabetes. In rare cases, magnesium supplements can be used for asthma, altitude sickness, chronic obstructive pulmonary disease (COPD) and Lyme disease.

Across the two genders, the older adults seem to have a lower level of magnesium compared to younger adults. This is caused by the inability of the gut to absorb magnesium as well as the kidney being unable to retain magnesium as you age. In case you suffer from type II diabetes, your kidney may excrete a lot of magnesium causing its deficit.

Do magnesium supplements work?

It's believed that supplementing with magnesium tablets can raise the level of magnesium in the blood serum and bones. The most effective form of magnesium supplements is those in the form of chloride, lactate, citrate, and aspartate. According to a number of research studies, people taking the supplements end up having more than the recommended daily allowance. The recommended amount of magnesium should be within 320-420 milligrams daily, which depends on the age or the activity.

Long-term studies have shown a connection between the high level of magnesium and a reduced risk of developing a heart disease, ischemic heart disease, stroke, and sudden cardiac death.

In about 7 studies that were done to more than 200, 000 participants, it was found that about 100 milligrams in excess magnesium daily can reduce your risk of stroke by around 8 percent. Though magnesium supplements are believed to lower hypertension, the effectiveness is not as it seems to be. Around 22 studies conducted on magnesium and hypertension found out that magnesium only managed to lower the pressure by 2-4 mmHg. Actually, hypertension can be as high with 20 mmHg, increasing from 140/90mmHg to 160/100 mmHg. The analysis to these studies indicated that hypertension was effectively addressed through an increase in magnesium content from fruits and veggies.

Supplements should offer at least 370 mg of magnesium daily to be effective, against the recommended 320 mg daily. Using of fruits and veggies also boosts the levels of other nutrients such as calcium or potassium. Thus, it is hard to determine independently how magnesium affects high blood pressure when the diet is used in place of supplements.

Type II diabetes is linked to low magnesium levels as deficiency of the mineral worsens insulin resistance, which results to unmonitored levels of blood sugar. However, insulin resistance can also cause a deficiency of magnesium, thus it's difficult to establish how the two affect each other. Diabetes may cause low levels of magnesium, which will cause the worsening of diabetes. On the other hand, magnesium supplements have shown potential in preventing migraine. However, a nutritional supplement butterbur is more advised for migraine prevention as compared to the use of magnesium.

More studies with the National Library of Medicine have found that magnesium supplements can help address pain from fibromyalgia and chronic fatigue syndrome. There's also evidence that they can assist in treating PMS, asthma attacks, hearing loss, kidney stones, high cholesterol and Chronic Obstructive Pulmonary Disease. However, there isn't enough studies to establish whether supplements may help address problems such as multiple sclerosis or Lyme disease, hay fever, ADHD, and anxiety.

Are the supplements safe?

Magnesium remains one of the 7 major elements required in the body, and its deficiency can pose serious problems among them death. On the other hand, taking in excess of one mineral can lead to a deficiency of another, where excessive magnesium generally causes a deficiency in calcium. It is quite hard to overdose magnesium from an ordinary diet, and overdose generally happens from laxatives or supplements.

If you suffer from kidney problems, you're more likely to face an overdose of magnesium. Consumption of magnesium to toxic levels can lead to symptoms such as diarrhea and stomach upsets, to other serious conditions like low blood pressure, slowed heart rate, confusion, and vomiting. A more severe overdose of magnesium can cause irregular heartbeat, coma, and problems in breathing or even death.

Additionally, magnesium supplements may interfere with other drugs among them antibiotics meant to address bacterial infections. The supplements can cause low absorption of antibiotics such as moxifloxacin and ciprofloxacin. The supplements are also counteractive on with osteoporosis drugs if taken too close, and can interfere with medications meant to address thyroid problems. Magnesium may also worsen the side effects of hypertension medications and raise the potency of diabetes medicines.

With all the information on magnesium, its deficiency and using diet and supplements to deal with deficiency, it is important to look at ways of addressing magnesium deficiency for long term health.

Eliminating Magnesium Deficiency For Long-Term Health And Longevity

Insufficient magnesium can lead to many health problems among them immune system depression, disrupted recovery and sleep, lack of energy, excess soreness, and muscle cramping. During intense activity, the deficiency can lead to fatal heart arrhythmias or irregular heartbeat. Magnesium is usually important in buffering the lactic acid and enhances uptake of oxygen and total work output. This reduces the heart rate and generation of carbon dioxide when doing tough exercises, and improves efficiency in cardiovascular activity.

Veggies, grains, nuts, and seeds can offer high amounts of magnesium, especially for active women. However, you can still be magnesium deficient even if you include these foods into the diets due to the combination of mineral loss through perspiration. Additionally, if you have an active lifestyle, you also face an accelerated mineral turn over that may cause depletion. In such cases, use of oral magnesium supplements may not completely deal with deficiency, as the amount of magnesium taken orally is not easily absorbed. Trying to take higher dosages of magnesium will definitely make the condition worse.

A better way of addressing deficiency of magnesium is through a technique referred as the transdermal application. Deficiency of magnesium can be addressed through the skin, a practice that is done in place of intravenous therapies. Applying magnesium through the skin can be effective in improving the absorption as the supplement travels through the gastrointestinal tract. The method also helps lower the metabolism of the drug by the liver and provides a more targeted application.

This method of application can also be used to deliver high dosages of precisely targeted magnesium supplement through the muscles before or after a workout. This treatment is aimed at boosting the performance and the recovery. As this transdermal magnesium bypasses the process of digestion, it's easier to achieve higher doses of the mineral as targeted. However, you need to monitor the amount of magnesium taken through transdermal delivery, as more than 500-1000 mg of magnesium can lead to health problems.

A way of using transdermal magnesium application is for instance trying an Epsom salt bath to deal with muscle soreness. Epsom salts deliver magnesium sulfate, to help address post workout recovery though more benefits can come from magnesium chloride crystals or flakes in the bath. Doing a magnesium chloride flake bath should deliver around 500mg of magnesium. In case you don't wish to hop into a full bath, you can as well soak your feet in magnesium chloride footbath especially after a long run or ride.

You can also enjoy benefits of topical magnesium that is also available as a form of spray, which you can use a number of sprays before workout. For instance, you can spray about 8-10 times on each arm, leg, or shoulders before a race or hard activity for longevity and optimal performance.

Therefore, your goal is to ensure that you take foods rich in magnesium, embrace supplementation, and topical use of magnesium for long term health and longevity.

CHAPTER 12: MAGNESIUM: A MIRACLE MINERAL?

What Is Magnesium And Why Do We Need It?

Magnesium is a mineral that is essential for life.

It is the fourth most common ion in your body, and the second most common ion in your cells. What does this mean? In a nutshell, your body cannot function without magnesium.

Magnesium regulates your blood pressure, keeps your heart healthy, builds strong bones, and keeps your cells and tissues in working order.

The Benefits Of Magnesium

Your health, your mood, your energy levels, even your sex life, are all dependent on the amount of magnesium you are giving your body! It is within your reach to quickly and easily impact your life in amazingly beneficial ways. Below are a few benefits of magnesium.

•   Increased energy

- Improved moods and decreased rates of depression and anxiety

- Better sleep

- Increased sex drive

- Lower inflammation levels

- Improved immune system

- Healthy blood pressure levels

- Improved cardiovascular health and lower risk of heart disease

- Strong bones and reduced risk of osteoporosis

- Reduced risk of developing Type II Diabetes

- Lower risk of hypertension

- Lower risk of chronic diseases

As you can see, the benefits of having the right amount of magnesium are substantial. Yet, experts claim that 75% of people are not meeting the minimum daily magnesium dietary requirements.

THIS SELF-ASSESSMENT CAN HELP DETERMINE YOUR RISK OF MAGNESIUM DEFICIENCY.

- I have trouble falling asleep or staying asleep (True/False)

- I have insomnia (True/False)

- I have muscle cramps or muscle tics (True/False)

- My muscles take a longer than average time to recover after exercise (True/False)

- I have muscle weakness (True/False)

- I have frequent diarrhea (True/False)

- I am frequently tired (True/False)

- I have a lot of stress in my life (True/False)

- I am diabetic (True/False)

- I take medication for heartburn (True/False)

- I take medication for diabetes, cancer, birth control, or asthma (True/False)

- I frequently take antibiotics (True/False)

- I take a calcium supplement that does not include magnesium (True/False)

143

- I have anxiety or depression (True/False)

- I eat a lot of processed foods, white flours, and sugars (True/False)

- I drink carbonated beverages (True/False)

- I drink more than 7 alcoholic beverages per week (True/False)

- My sex drive is low (True/False)

- I am over 55 (True/False)

Total # of True Responses:

How did you do?

Each of these factors are contributors to or signs of magnesium deficiency. If you selected more than 3, you are at risk for magnesium deficiency. If you selected any factor and are older than 55, you are at an even greater risk of magnesium deficiency, as magnesium absorption decreases as you age.

Likewise, as 75% of the population does not meet magnesium intake requirements, you will likely find benefit from the information in this book.

Why Are So Many Of Us Deficient In Magnesium?

The rate of magnesium deficiency in the first world is astounding. Why is magnesium deficiency so widespread, even with supplementation and healthy diets?

Here are a few reasons for magnesium deficiency:

• DEPLETION OF MINERALS IN FOOD SUPPLY DUE TO MODERN FARMING PRACTICES

o A 2004 study found that the levels of minerals in food has declined significantly since 1950.

o What does this mean? If you are eating the same foods as your parents or grandparents did in 1950, you are getting significantly less vitamins and minerals. You likely can't get all the magnesium you need from food alone.

• INCREASED CONSUMPTION OF PROCESSED FOODS OVER WHOLE FOODS.

o Processing foods completely eliminates or significantly reduces magnesium content.

• TAKING CERTAIN MEDICATIONS INCLUDING MEDICATIONS THAT TREAT ACID REFLUX, DIABETES, CANCER, ANTIBIOTICS, AND MORE.

- HAVING A GI DISORDER THAT HINDERS DIGESTION AND ABSORPTION.

- HAVING DIABETES.

- HAVING A KIDNEY DISEASE.

- DRINKING MORE THAN 7 ALCOHOLIC BEVERAGES PER WEEK.

- DRINKING CARBONATED BEVERAGES FREQUENTLY.

- IF YOU ARE OLDER THAN 55.

- IF YOU TAKE A CALCIUM SUPPLEMENT THAT DOES NOT ALSO INCLUDE MAGNESIUM.

- HAVING SIGNIFICANT OR PROLONGED STRESS IN YOUR LIFE.

As you can see, there are many factors that can contribute to magnesium deficiency. Even if you meet the daily recommended intake of magnesium, you may have other factors that stop your body from absorbing magnesium (such as GI difficulties, age, medication, or stress).

Magnesium deficiency is extremely common. However, it is underdiagnosed. 50% of people with magnesium deficiency that are screened, are not diagnosed. Modern testing methods are not able to accurately determine magnesium levels, as the majority (99%) of magnesium is stored in the body's bones, muscles and soft tissue. Because of this, it is more reliable to determine magnesium deficiency by relying on clinical presentation or symptoms.

The following is a list of symptoms that are found in magnesium deficiency. However, sometimes magnesium deficiency has no symptoms. It's not until a person develops a disease due to, or correlated with, magnesium deficiency like osteoporosis or heart disease that the problem of low magnesium is discovered.

Common Symptoms:

• FACIAL, EYE OR MUSCLE TICS

• MUSCLE SPASMS AND MUSCLE CRAMPS

• Depression

• Anxiety

• Insomnia

• PALPITATIONS OR IRREGULAR/RAPID HEART RATE

• WEAKNESS AND FATIGUE

• Migraines

- Nausea

- IMPAIRED COGNITIVE FUNCTION

- LOW SEX DRIVE

You may not have any symptoms related to magnesium deficiency. However, as mentioned you may develop or have a condition related to chronic magnesium deficiency. These conditions can include:

- MOOD DISORDERS: DEPRESSION AND ANXIETY

- SLEEP DISORDERS: INSOMNIA

- CHRONIC PAIN: MIGRAINES, CLUSTER HEADACHES, NEURALGIA, FIBROMYALGIA

- BONE HEALTH: OSTEOPEROSIS, OSTEOPENIA, OSTEOARTHRITIS

- FEMALE HEALTH: PMS, PCOS, MENOPAUSE, DYSMENORRHEA, INFERTILITY

- HEART HEALTH: HYPERTENSION, AND CARDIOVASCULAR DISEASE

- TYPE II DIABETES

- BRAIN HEALTH: DEMENTIA AND ALZHEIMER'S DISEASE

In the next chapters, we'll look at how your magnesium levels impact your mood, your sleep, your health, and your sex drive.

Let's get started.

The Science Behind How Magnesium Can Boost Your Mood

Magnesium has a huge impact on your mood. Why?

First, because magnesium deficiency causes a decrease in your brain's serotonin levels. Serotonin regulates your mood. This includes happiness, sadness, fear and anxiety. Too little serotonin is linked to depression. Low levels of magnesium lead to low levels of serotonin which leads to depression, sadness, and greater levels of fear and anxiety. (For more information, you can read 2017 study about magnesium's effect on stress and anxiety, or a 2013 study on magnesium in depression.)

Second, magnesium regulates the fight or flight response by deactivating the NMDA receptor in the brain (calcium and glutamate activate it). If Magnesium is not there to deactivate the receptor or prevent it from activating then your brain's stress response is increased, your neurons are damaged, and cell death can occur.

Finally, magnesium regulates your brain's stress response by preventing the release of stress hormones - including cortisol. (For more on this mechanism read this 2002 study by Murck). Magnesium also prevents stress hormones from entering the brain.

The bottom line: magnesium deficiency is related to depression, anxiety, chronic stress, fear, sadness, and chronic raised levels of stress hormones - a known contributor to inflammation and disease.

The Good News

All the studies showing low magnesium leading to depression and anxiety have a flip side. Magnesium supplementation boosts mood, increases feelings of happiness, calmness and well-being, and soothes your body/brain in times of stress.

Magnesium supplementation has also been shown to reduce anxiety and increase mental well-being. (See this 2017 study by Boyle et al)

Magnesium supplementation has been shown to be as effective as anti-depressant medication in mild depression, and faster-acting than anti-depressant medication. In cases of more severe depression, magnesium supplementation increases the effectiveness of anti-depressant medication. (For more information, read this fascinating randomized double blind placebo control 2017 study by Rajizadeh et al.; and this medical review and hypothesis by Eby III et al)

Even in people who are not depressed, and not particularly anxious, magnesium boosts happiness, well-being and calmness. Magnesium is nature's way of helping us deal with the stress of everyday life. You don't need to have depression or anxiety to reap the benefits of magnesium – it will boost your mood and reduce feelings of stress regardless of where you are starting. If you are stressed, it will reduce your stress. If you are happy, it can boost your happiness even more. Magnesium is a win/win for your happiness quotient.

The Science Behind How Magnesium Can Cure Insomnia

Insomnia and sleep trouble effect millions of people, as does magnesium deficiency.

Not having enough magnesium has been shown to cause insomnia. Lack of magnesium has also been shown to cause light and restless sleep – keeping people from going having a deep and rejuvenating night sleep. On top of this, magnesium supplementation has been shown to cure insomnia due to restless leg syndrome. Could lack of magnesium be the cause of your sleep troubles? (See Boonsma, Abbasi et al., and Hornyak for reviews on magnesium's role in insomnia).

If you suffer from insomnia or difficulty sleeping – you are not alone. The National Institute of Health says that thirty percent (30%) of the population suffers from sleep disruption and more than fifty percent (50%) of older adults have insomnia (See Abbasi, 2012)

As you read in the previous chapter, Magnesium reduces stress and increases calm. Magnesium has been shown in studies to increase the activity of the parasympathetic nervous system (See this study by Wienecke 2016). The parasympathetic nervous system slows the heart rate and relaxes muscles. Magnesium also helps regulate neurotransmitters, including GABA. When magnesium increases the activity of GABA receptors, it reduces anxiety and calms nerves. (For more about GABA and magnesium read this 2008 study by Poleszak) This mechanism, activating GABA, is what popular over-the-counter sleep medications use. However, you can get the same effect, with more benefits and less side effects, using magnesium.

The bottom line: magnesium deficiency can cause insomnia, and sleep disruption. Magnesium supplementation causes a similar mechanism as popular over the counter sleep medications to improve sleep.

The Good News

If you have insomnia, trouble falling asleep, trouble falling back to sleep, restless leg syndrome induced insomnia, or a lack of deep restful sleep, then supplementing with magnesium can alleviate all of these problems. Even if you get a good night's sleep, magnesium can help you fall asleep faster, have a deeper, more prolonged sleep, less night awakenings, less early morning awakenings, and a higher production of sleep hormones (See Abbasi). All of these benefits have been proven in medical studies.

Lack of sleep has been shown to increase your risk for obesity, heart disease, diabetes, high blood pressure and infections. Lack of sleep has also been shown to decrease testosterone and sex drive. Insomnia can also harm your critical thinking skills, and memory and cognition.

Insomnia also prevents your skin and tissues from healing and causes more wrinkles.

Again, the good news is that magnesium has been shown to be incredibly effective at curing insomnia, deepening sleep, and preventing sleep difficulties – leading to a more restful, beneficial night's sleep.

The Science Behind How Magnesium Can Prevent Illness

Magnesium is truly a miracle mineral. It is necessary for more than 300 metabolic reactions in your body. It also functions to regulate energy production, nutrient uptake, blood glucose control, blood pressure, muscle and nerve communication, DNA and RNA synthesis, and controls countless more functions in your body. If you don't have enough magnesium, these functions can suffer, and disease can take root.

There are dozens of diseases that are associated with chronic magnesium deficiency. Let's look at a few now.

Type II Diabetes:

Low magnesium intake is associated with the development of Type II Diabetes. Studies have shown that increasing the intake of magnesium can reduce the risk of developing Type II Diabetes. (See Larsson et al 2007) One study showed that increasing the dietary magnesium intake to RDA recommended levels significantly improved insulin resistance. It has also been shown that magnesium supplementation can reduce the risk of progressing from pre-diabetes to actual diabetes by reducing plasma glucose levels.

The bottom line: if you are at risk of developing Type II Diabetes, or have pre-diabetes, increasing your magnesium intake can help reduce your risk, or prevent you from developing Type II Diabetes.

High Blood Pressure And Heart Attack:

Magnesium deficiency is one of the leading causes of heart disease.

Your magnesium intake has a direct effect on your body's ability to regulate your blood pressure. Magnesium effects your body's vascular smooth muscle cells relaxation ability and the ratio of sodium/potassium to calcium – which has a direct impact on blood pressure control.

Interestingly, many people are treated with blood pressure medications that deplete the body of magnesium. When they are given magnesium supplementation in conjunction with these medications, their blood pressure reduces significantly. (See Saito et al)

In people with mild or borderline hypertension, magnesium supplementation returns blood pressure to normal. In people with hypertension, magnesium supplementation for more than 3 weeks has shown significant benefit to diastolic blood pressure.

Long-term follow-up studies have also shown people with magnesium intakes higher than the RDA (recommended daily allowances) have anywhere from a 40-77% reduced risk of cardiac death.

The bottom line: by increasing your magnesium intake, you can significantly reduce your risk for heart disease. This is because magnesium improves heart muscles, regulates your blood pressure, and improves your blood flow. It reduces blood pressure, steadies your heart rhythm, decreases inflammation, and reduces blood clotting.

Migraine Headaches:

It has been shown that people with migraines and cluster headaches are frequently deficient in magnesium. Evidence shows that supplementing with magnesium for 9 weeks reduces migraine frequency by nearly half. Use of magnesium during a migraine, also has been shown to reduce symptoms and duration.

The bottom line: if you suffer from headaches or migraines, supplementation with magnesium will be beneficial in reducing migraine frequency.

Alzheimer's Disease And Dementia:

Researchers have not determined why magnesium plays a role in Alzheimer's Disease and dementia. However, it has been found that magnesium stores are depleted in people with Alzheimer's Disease and treatment with magnesium improves memory in people with mild and moderate dementia and Alzheimer's Disease. Magnesium supplementation has also been found to reduce the plaque that forms in the brain in Alzheimer's and even prevent memory decline.

Memory and cognition have also been shown to improve with magnesium supplementation. If you want to improve your day to day mental function, then increasing your magnesium is an excellent route. Magnesium enhances learning and memory function in both young and old. Supplementation increases the brain's functioning synapses, improves brain signals, and benefits brain processes that are crucial for both long and short-term memory.

Magnesium has also been shown to improve learning abilities, with magnesium supplementation speeding learning and increasing recall.

The bottom line: if you want to decrease your risk of Alzheimer's and dementia, and improve your cognitive function and memory, magnesium is key.

Osteoporosis And Osteoarthritis

Magnesium is crucial for bone health and the prevention of osteoporosis and osteoarthritis. Magnesium deficiency directly contributes to osteoporosis. Magnesium deficiency has been linked to osteoporosis and higher magnesium status prevents bone loss. In numerous studies the supplementation of magnesium in women with osteoporosis has resulted in a reduction in fractures and a significant increase in bone density.

Magnesium intake is as important as calcium intake in the health of bones. Intake of magnesium directly impacts the amount of bone children have – regardless of the amount of calcium intake.

Magnesium also has an impact on osteoarthritis. Magnesium is responsible for making sure that calcium stays in the bone. When magnesium is chronically low or deficient osteoarthritis is at risk of developing. In fact, the risk of developing osteoarthritis increases as magnesium intake decreases. Magnesium has also been shown to be useful in treating osteoarthritis as it has a significant protective effect on cartilage tissue and bone health.

The bottom line: increasing your magnesium intake can prevent and even treat osteoporosis and osteoarthritis.

The Science Behind How Magnesium Can Improve Your Sex Drive

Low sex drive effects nearly 45% of women and more than 30% of men. Studies have shown that people with higher circulating or free testosterone have higher sex drive – and magnesium is directly related to the level of free testosterone in your body.

Magnesium is key in the production of sex hormones – testosterone, estrogen, progesterone, and brain chemicals that regulate sex drive. Low levels of magnesium result in low sex hormones. In both women and men, testosterone is key to sex drive.

As women age, estrogen decreases, as does testosterone. It is the decrease in testosterone in both men and women that actually causes a decrease in libido. Increasing magnesium increases free and total testosterone levels. Magnesium prevents testosterone from binding to proteins, which increases your level of free testosterone. This in turn will give you a higher sex drive.

Other factors that contribute to low sex drive including stress, anxiety, depression, and lower testosterone with aging can all be improved with magnesium.

The bottom line: magnesium increases free testosterone, which increases your sex drive. This is why magnesium is so helpful in boosting sex drive in both men and women.

The Good News

If you suffer from a reduced sex drive or a low libido, supplementing with magnesium can boost your sex drive at the cellular and hormonal level. It won't take long for the effects of magnesium to kick in, and for you to start experiencing the benefits of increased testosterone and a higher sex drive.

You have learned that magnesium has immense benefits for your health, happiness, sex drive and long-term well-being. If you have symptoms of magnesium deficiency you will benefit from the magnesium cure. If you suspect you have adequate magnesium levels, you can still benefit from the effects of magnesium – as shown in countless studies – people with adequate magnesium intake still benefit from increasing magnesium levels.

This chapter will walk you through how to use magnesium for noticeable benefit in 7 days or less.

How Much Magnesium Do I Need?

The RDA for women is 310mg per day for women ages 19-30, and 320mg per day for women 31 years and older. If a woman is breastfeeding the recommendation increases to 350mg per day for ages 19-30, and 360mg per day for ages 31 and over.

The RDA for men ages 19-30 is 400mg per day, and 420mg per day for men ages 31 and up.

How Long Will It Take To Feel Better?

In terms of insomnia, sleep difficulties, muscle pain and exercise recovery, and mood, magnesium's effects can be noticed after the first dose.

Within seven days you will notice a greater effect on your levels of calm, happiness, sleep quality, libido, and overall feelings of well-being.

If you supplement with magnesium long-term, you will receive the amazing long-term benefits of reduced risk of Type II Diabetes, Osteoporosis and Osteoarthritis, Alzheimer's and dementia, and cardiovascular disease. Likewise, increasing magnesium intake can help reverse pre-diabetes, osteoporosis, and mild hypertension.

Types Of Supplementation

As mentioned previously, it is difficult to get the necessary magnesium from diet alone. However, eating a diet rich in magnesium foods can still be extremely helpful in increasing your magnesium status. The appendix has a list of the top magnesium rich foods, and recipes. Too start, it is recommended that you use a combined approach of incorporating magnesium rich foods in your daily diet and using transdermal magnesium.

Note: Oral magnesium supplements have a limited absorption rate of 4-50% and common side effects including GI discomfort and diarrhea. For this reason, transdermal magnesium is recommended over oral magnesium supplements.

Transdermal Magnesium:

The best way to quickly and effectively increase your magnesium is through topical or transdermal application. The topical application allows the magnesium to be directly absorbed at the cellular level, without the side effects or limited absorption of oral supplementation.

Epsom Salts (Magnesium Sulfate) or bath salts (Magnesium Chloride) are the first-line method of topical application, as bath flakes are the most inexpensive method, very safe, and proven in scientific studies to be effective in increasing magnesium levels.

Magnesium can also be applied topically through:

- Magnesium Oil

- Magnesium Gel

- Magnesium Lotion

The studies show that daily application of transdermal magnesium significantly increases the level of serum magnesium. Studies have also shown that a mere 2-3 Epsom salt baths a week have significant impact on cardiovascular health.

Bath Flakes Routine:

- Begin by adding 1-3 cups of Epsom salts to a foot bath or bath of warm (not hot) water.

- Soak for 30 minutes.

- Soak every day for 7 days.

- After the first week, complete 2-3 soaks per week.

Magnesium Oil Spray Routine:

Alternatively, you may prefer to use magnesium oil or lotion supplementation.

If you prefer to use lotions, gels, or oils, apply the product to your legs, arms and torso – avoid your face, sensitive areas, and mucous membranes. Apply the product amount recommended on the product instructions. You may experience tingling, or a residue. After 20 minutes, wipe off the product with a damp washcloth.

You may make your own Magnesium Oil, or Magnesium Lotion with the following recipes.

Magnesium Oil Recipe:

1 cup of filtered water

1 cup of Magnesium Chloride (bath flakes)

Bring the water to a boil in a non-aluminum pan. Turn off the burner. Add the magnesium chloride and stir until dissolved. Cool. Pour into a spray bottle.

For use, spray 1-3 spritzes in your hand and rub into legs, arms, or torso. There may be tingling, and a residue. After 20 minutes, wipe off with a damp cloth.

Limit oil application to no more than 3 spritzes per day.

Magnesium Lotion Recipe:

1 cup of body lotion or body butter

2 Tbsp of Magnesium Oil

Use a hand mixer to mix magnesium oil and lotion on medium speed for 2 minutes. Once thoroughly blended, put lotion in opaque container.

Apply a small amount (equivalent to one pump) to legs, arms, or torso. Tingling and residue may occur. Wipe off with damp cloth after 20 minutes.

Limit lotion application to no more than 1 pump per day.

Daily Intake of Magnesium Rich Foods:

As well as supplementing with topical applications of magnesium, you should include magnesium rich foods in your diet.

Top Magnesium Rich Foods To Include In Your Diet:

Spinach (156mg in 1 cup)

Swiss Chard (150 mg in 1 cup)

Beat Greens (100 mg in 1 cup)

Roasted Almonds (96 mg in ¼ cup)

Roasted Pumpkin Seeds (163 mg in ¼ cup)

Cashews (120mg in ¼ cup)

Sesame Seeds (125mg in ¼ cup)

Sunflower Seeds (115 in ¼ cup)

Sunflower Seed Butter (101 mg in 2 Tbsp)

Almond Butter (90 mg in 2 Tbsp)

Dark Chocolate (64 mg in 1 ounce)

Soybeans (150 mg in 1 cup)

Black Beans (120 mg in 1 cup)

Navy Beans (100 mg in 1 cup)

Pinto Beans (85 mg in 1 cup)

Tofu (65 mg in ½ cup)

Quinoa (160 mg in 1 cup)

Brown Rice (85 mg in 1 cup)

Oatmeal (140 mg in 1 cup uncooked oats)

*Note: Magnesium content will vary in foods based on growing conditions and soil. The reported content of magnesium in foods varies between reporting sources based on food tests. The numbers provided are estimates. Also, remember, the amount of magnesium your body absorbs from food depends upon your body and your personal gastrointestinal health (for example, people with low stomach acid absorb less magnesium).

A Word Of Caution

Consult with your physician before beginning magnesium supplementation or a new diet. Magnesium intake from supplements exceeding 350 mg per day may cause adverse side effects including: diarrhea, nausea, vomiting, irregular heartbeat, low blood pressure, confusion, slowed breathing, coma, and death (note that this warning does not include magnesium intake from food, as the body naturally excretes any excess magnesium from food in the urine). These side effects are rare. Do not exceed recommended amounts of supplementation. Also, consult with your physician on any interactions magnesium supplementation may have with medication you take. Ask your physician about any effects magnesium supplementation may have on any medical condition you have. People with kidney disease, or impaired kidney function should not supplement with magnesium. Consult with your doctor before magnesium supplementation if you have: kidney disease, diabetes, excessively slow heart rate, myasthenia gravis, bowel obstruction, or are taking antibiotics, blood pressure medication, blood thinners, thyroid medication, or medication for osteoporosis.

APPENDIX

Magnesium Cure Smoothie: (Serves 1)

Throw together in a blender and blend until smooth:

1Tbsp flax seed (55mg)

2 Tbsp sunflower seed butter (101mg)

¾ cup soft tofu (80mg) or 1 cup of yogurt (47mg)

1 banana (32mg)

1 square (1 oz) 80% (or higher) dark chocolate (64mg)

1 cup cow milk (27mg) or 1 cup soy milk (61mg)

1 cup of ice (optional)

Total magnesium: 326mg – 393mg

Magnesium Cure Snack Mix: (Serves 1)

Combine:

¼ cup roasted pumpkin seeds (163mg)

3 ounces of dark chocolate chips (123mg)

¼ cup whole almonds (96mg)

3 oz banana chips (65mg)

1.5 oz (small box) raisins (14mg)

Total Magnesium: 461mg

Magnesium Cure Spinach Soup: (Serves 2)

1 pound frozen spinach (396mg)

2 cups of milk or cream (54mg)

1 medium onion (11mg)

2-4 garlic cloves

3 Tbsp almond butter (135mg)

1 oz slivered almonds (76mg)

1 Tbsp lemon juice

Salt and pepper to taste

Total Magnesium: 672mg

Add 2Tbsp of oil to pan and cook minced onion and garlic until translucent. Add spinach and 1 cup of cream or milk. Use immersion blender and blend until smooth. Add almond butter, lemon juice and salt and pepper and mix thoroughly. Add slivered almonds as garnish. Serve.

Magnesium Cure Tacos: (Serves 2)

1 cup canned black beans (120 mg)

1 cup tofu (130 mg)

Chili powder, oregano, garlic

1 medium onion, diced (11 mg)

1 cup brown rice (85 mg)

1 avocado, mashed (58 mg)

1 cup shredded cheddar cheese (32 mg)

6 corn taco shells (17mg per shell)

Salsa

Total Magnesium 572mg

Begin by cooking brown rice, to equal 1 cup cooked. Follow package directions.

While the rice cooks prepare the tofu and beans.

Add 1 Tbsp oil to pan, add minced onion and garlic, cook until translucent, add diced tofu and cook until brown, remove from heat.

In a saucepan, cook on low, canned black beans, dash of chili powder, oregano, salt and pepper to taste.

When all ingredients are cooked, prepare the tacos.

Scoop into corn taco shells:

- Bottom layer brown rice.

- Next layer tofu.

- Next layer black beans.

- Next layer avocado.

- Next layer salsa.

- Top layer cheese.

- Serve and enjoy.

If you follow a day of eating these recipes for breakfast, lunch, snack and dinner you will have a total magnesium intake of 1476mg! That is more than 3 times the daily recommended value for men, and more than 4 times the daily recommended value for women. If you only have the smoothie or the trail mix, you will meet your daily requirement. Which, as you may recall, 75% of the population fails to meet on a daily basis.

Combine these foods with your topical magnesium supplementation and you will be on your way to reaping the extraordinary benefits of magnesium.

CHAPTER 13: SYMPTOMS & CAUSES OF LOW MAGNESIUM

IN THE BODY

In this chapter, we will discuss symptoms of low magnesium in the body. If you are having any of these symptoms mention here, then your body is low on magnesium.

• Anxiety

• Impaired memory

• High blood pressure (Hypertension)

• Depression

• Behavioral disturbances

• Lethargy

• Chronic back pain

• Headaches

• Migraines

• Muscular pain

• Insomnia

• Muscles cramps

- Constipation

- Brain Fog

- Tension

- ADHD

- Tendonitis

- Anger

- Aggression

- Anxiety disorders such as OCD and many more.

So if you are suffering or

experiencing any of these symptoms, then you need to start eating magnesium-

rich food, or supplements to improve your health condition.

Magnesium deficiency is found in 80% of heart attack, and this makes it essential m ineral in the cardiovascular function beca use calcium controls the contraction of the heart while magnesium controls the relaxation of the heart and magnesium clears out calcium so that you can relax.

With this, you can see that magnesium is a super mineral for the body.

Causes of Magnesium deficient in the body

Diet: Many people in today's world are so obsessed with fast food that they consume less leafy greens which are the primary source of magnesium, and also magnesium can be found in nuts and seeds but mainly in leafy greens.

Stress: This is another way the body gets depleted of magnesium because our body uses magnesium to deal with stress and that is why it is essential to eat healthy food, exercise, and sleep when you are going through stressful times.

Alcohol: Alcohol acts intensely as a magnesium diuretic which leads to an

increase in the urinary excretion from the body. With an excessive intake of alcohol and development of alcoholism, stored magnesium in the body is depleted along with other electrolytes.

A little awareness has been paid to the important value of magnesium. As a preventive measure to minimize the deleterious effects of excessive use of alcohol or to prevent the growth of cancer that can occur if precautions necessary to be taken is overlooked or ignored.

Drug depletion: if you're on proton pump inhibitors whether it's prevacid, omeprazole or Nexium and all the PPI medications that lower stomach acid, is

a

great

chance

you're

causing

nutritional deficiencies with that family of drugs and also the medications that are used to treat high blood pressure they actually create magnesium deficiency in the body. So many people are developing magnesium deficiencies because of the overuse of some antibiotics such as ciprofloxacin for urinary tract infection. It is essential to take magnesium supplements or eat rich magnesium foods to avoid magnesium depletion in the body.

Karen's health deteriorated so much over the use of ciprofloxacin antibiotic in treating urinary tract infection, she was on an antibiotic for so long, and this led to vast depletion of magnesium in her body which took her several years to get her health back. In her words, "The antibiotic I took did a lot of damage to my gut and immune system because I needed a fast cure."

Heavy antibiotic use has been shown to promote and multiply yeasts that live in our digestive system and what this yeast does is that it get stuck in our digestive wall and this can lead to leaky gut.

Every time you eat food, what you are eating is leaking into your bloodstream, and that is not good because of your immune system start looking at these foreign

objects,

and

it

gets

overwhelmed and stressed out because it knows that it's not supposed to be there and this is how inflammations start happening, and we end up getting

sick. When you have a leaky gut, it is very hard to absorb the nutrients in the food you are eating.

MAGNESIUM AND

DEPRESSION

A lot of our health issues can be solved just

by

adding

a

magnesium

supplement or eating lots of foods that contain a high level of

magnesium.

Magnesium is involved in so many functions in the body and brain; it is used by so many different mechanisms, and if you lack magnesium in your body, that alone can trigger extreme low

mood

or

even depression. I have heard stories o f people who overcame depression and depressed mood by adding magnesium supplements to their diet.

Magnesium deficiency is what most people lack today. The relaxing and calming effects found in magnesium helps to relax the body and improve our sleep mood which helps combat depression or even anxiety. So if you are suffering from depression, it is now time to get on those leafy green food and eliminate processed food from your diet

if

you

want

to

overcome

depression. With this, you will see how the food we eat plays a significant role in our overall well being.

The food you consume that are low in magnesium are the key things that are affecting your mood which eventually leads to depression. Sometimes after working out in the gym or had a stressful day, I take my organic

magnesium supplement because I know it will relax my muscles and reduce my stress level. I am a big fan of magnesium I take it every day and eat foods and nuts that are rich in magnesium.

NMDA

Receptor

is

receptors in your brain, and they play a role in neuroplasticity. Abnormal NM

DA function plays a role in depression.

So if your NMDA receptors are not functioning properly, what can help it work properly is magnesium because it's an NMDA regulator. Some studies have shown that higher intake of magnesium supplements at baseline are associated with better responses to any depressants.

A test was carried out on people who suffered

from

treatment-resistant

depression and supplemented them with magnesium, and what they found out

was

that

supplementing

magnesium

with

antidepressants

worked perfectly for such individuals.

Research has found out that low magnesium level in the body can lead to depression. If you want to enhance your magnesium intake, like when you feel your diet is low in this beneficial substance or other certain essential minerals and vitamins, then you have to consume more fruits and vegetable as much as you can.

You can even drink mineral water, for me. I like San Pellegrino it is full of essential minerals that you can drink.

When your body needs those vital minerals, it will extract them from your body that is the more reason you have to give your body the essential minerals to work with.

For instance, imagine what will happen if you mistakenly fill a Diesel in a Petrol car it will clog your fuel filter and then damage your fuel injector, the same thing happen to our bodies when you are feeding the body with the wrong nutrients it will lead to more complications.

Before you run to the supplement store or think that low magnesium level is the cause of your depression. Listen, get your diet in check, and then see how that helps you. If it makes you feel better, then okay, but if you are suffering from depression or have taken an antidepressant; my

advice is to consult your doctor immed iately, and see if he can test your magnesium level, as that might help in solving your problem.

MAGNESIUM AND

MIGRAINES

Migraines are very popular today, as millions of people around the globe are suffering from a migraine headache. It is a debilitating condition because they can't focus at work, play with their kids or even get out of bed, so we are looking for a natural solution and magnesium is a significant first step.

CONCLUSION

I have come to the end of the book and I really have to say, I am sure so are you. Not only has this book enabled me to give knowledge, but it has also given me more knowledge than that I had when I began writing. The research has been enlightening and I now know even more about the miracle that is this mineral than the miracle I thought it was in the beginning. The importance of this mineral to the body is so intricate that it can never be extricated.

The book gently propels you through everything that you possibly need to know about magnesium. It goes through what magnesium is and why it should hold that special place in our lives. It explains about some of the many symptoms of magnesium deficiency, explaining about ALL the symptoms would require a stand-alone book about magnesium deficiency symptoms. It is that serious. The book goes on to explain about the signs in your body that can tell you that you are running on magnesium low. The life or death uses of magnesium in the ER are also highlighted, together with other medical but not ER uses of magnesium.

To cut a very long story short, the book gives you all the insights into the uses of the mineral, where you can get it and how, ways you can improve your body stocks of the mineral and also talks about some things we do which limit the uses of magnesium in our bodies. It is comprehensive and I believe you will enjoy reading it as you are catapulted into the realm of magnesium use and not abuse. You will surely enjoy life and much better health as you practice what the book says.

www.ingramcontent.com/pod-product-compliance
Lightning Source LLC
Chambersburg PA
CBHW060330030426
42336CB00011B/1274